P9-AGP-446

DATE DUE

JE 1 0 '94			
OC 1 4 '94			
DE 9 '94			
MR 1 0 95			
NO 2 5 '96			
AP 3 0 '97			

DEMCO 38-296

THE HIGH PERFORMANCE HEART

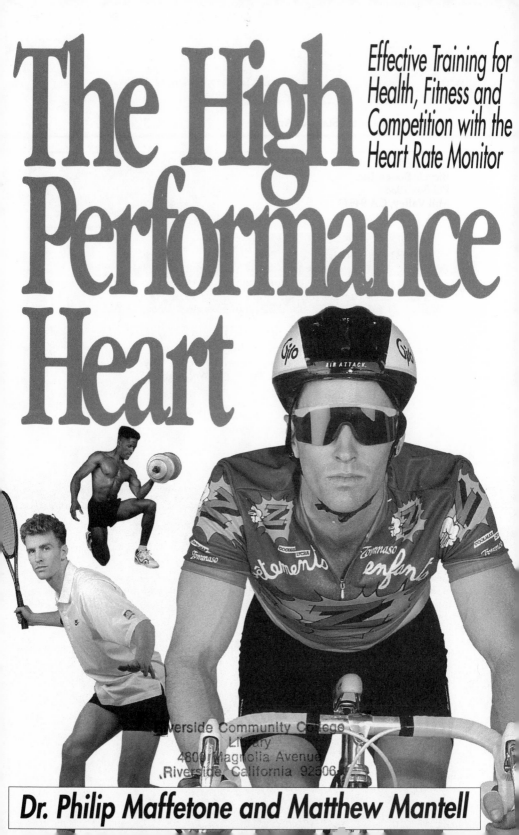

Copyright © Philip B. Maffetone and Matthew E. Mantell, 1991

RC1236.H43 M34 1991
Maffetone, Philip.
The high performance heart
effective training for
health, fitness, and
competition with the heart
```` ```````

Distributed to the book trade by:
USA: The Talman Company, New York (until Dec 1991)
         National Book Network, Lanham, MD (effective January 1992)
Canada: Raincoast Book Distribution, Vancouver, BC
UK: Chris Lloyd Sales and Marketing Services, Poole, Dorset

Cover: Design and photographs by Kent Lytle
         Bicycle and cycling dress courtesy A Bicycle Odyssey, Sausalito
         Tennis dress courtesy Love-30, San Anselmo

Cataloging in Publication Data
Maffetone, Philip B. and Matthew E. Mantell,
The High Performance Heart, Effective training for competition, health
and fitness with the heart rate monitor.
Bibliography: p. Includes index.
1. Health and fitness
2. Sports, training — manuals, handbooks, etc.
3. Bicycles and bicycling — manuals, handbooks, etc.
4. Heart rate monitor
5. Authorship
I. Title

Library of Congress Catalog Card No. 91-73663

ISBN 0-933201-37-0, Paperback original
````

To Lillian
M.E.M

_____ To everybody pursuing both health *and* fitness

P.M.

"I use the heart rate monitor everyday in training, and on the bike during the Ironman race. It allows me to be more precise, prevent injury and raise my performance."

— **Mark Allen**, '89 and '90 Ironman winner

"The heart rate monitor has been my training companion for years. Without it, I'd still be injured and would not have the success I now enjoy."

— **Colleen Cannon**, Triathlon Champion

"The pulse rate provides the most readily obtainable and concrete data about an athlete's fitness. As a result, the heart rate monitor is an essential tool for a cyclist."

— **Alexander Kuznetsov**, coach of the Leningrad-based LocoSphinx club and the Soviet amateur team at the '91 Tour Du Pont.

ACKNOWLEDGEMENTS

For her tireless research assistance, we owe thanks to Kathryn Silberger, Librarian at Marist College in Poughkeepsie, New York. Also, we are extremely grateful for the editorial help and support provided by Rob van der Plas, our editor at Bicycle Books. A special tip of the bike cap goes to Jonathan Sternfield, a longtime friend and co-conspirator.

FOREWORD

by Massimo Testa MD
Physician to the Motorola bicycle racing team, director of the Milan Sport Medicine Research Center

When Andy Hampsten won the hardest uphill time trial of the 1988 Giro d'Italia, he became the first American overall winner in the race's history. Many observers were intrigued by the flexible strap that was visible under his aerodynamic skin suit: They later learned he was wearing a heart rate monitor to keep track of his physical performance.

At that time, the use of a heart rate monitor was still quite uncommon, even in professional bicycle racing circles. Since then, what was once a novelty has become a widely used tool in competition and training. In fact, most top athletes and their coaches have discovered that the heart rate monitor is the ideal instrument to increase the efficiency of the athlete's training and competitive effort.

Now, at last, here is the book that shows the 'ordinary' amateur athlete how to get the same benefits as the professionals on the major teams. This book by my friends Dr. Philip Maffetone and Matthew Mantell explains how to effectively use the heart rate monitor for effective training, whether for fitness and competition. In a logical step-by-step process it explains how to go about choosing the equipment and how to use it to maximum advantage. It develops all the important aspects of scientific training methods to achieve a personalized training program based on the use of the HRM. I am sure this book will help you improve your athletic performance while maximizing health and fitness.

Through my experience as a physician to professional bicycle racing teams, I have become convinced that the heart rate is the most precise parameter to evaluate an athlete's physical performance outside the physiology laboratory. The heart rate monitor provides the accurate and instantaneous feedback that allows the informed and intelligent athlete to optimize his or her efforts, whether training for competition or fitness.

Working with both amateur and professional endurance athletes has convinced me that the subjective feeling of fatigue is not always an accurate index for developing an optimal, personalized training program. The heart rate, on the other hand, is a valuable and objective means of determining the athlete's responses and adaptations to every workload situation. It also helps test the athlete's aerobic efficiency under different conditions, providing valuable information to establish the most effective training techniques, the most efficient riding style or to fine-tune your equipment.

For the recreational athlete, the heart rate monitor can also be an invaluable source of information. It prevents 'weekend warriors' (those who don't have time to train on a regular basis) from exceeding their limits, thus endangering their health in pursuit of fitness.

For exercise programs dealing with cardiac rehabilitation or weight reduction, the capability to monitor the workout level is very important. Patients recovering from a heart attack or heart surgery can maintain the target zone recommended by their cardiologist. Overweight patients adhering to a regimen of proper diet and aerobic exercise can use the heart rate monitor during their long, steady workout sessions to make sure they are metabolizing fats.

Clearly, the heart rate monitor has the potential to revolutionize training for health, fitness and competition. I can't emphasize enough how important it is to get a correct understanding of the subject across to athletes and fitness conscious people everywhere. The authors of *The High Performance Heart* have done an excellent job of demystifying the subject, thus putting a very important tool into your hands. I am confident this book will prove invaluable to all who strive for fitness and health.

Table of Contents

INTRODUCTION

Today, training and competing in virtually all athletic disciplines has become quite systematic, if not truly scientific. This is a far cry from the not so distant past when folklore and tradition prevailed.

One quaint custom held by many coaches and trainers in the 1950's was that athletes should never drink water during their workouts. To do so, in their opinion, would sap a player's mental toughness. Even when temperatures broke the century mark, the water bucket appeared only after practice. Burly football players were not the only athletes forced to adhere to this convention. It was also applied to whippet-like long distance runners. As late as the 1976 Olympic Games, there was a rule prohibiting the consumption of any fluids during the first six miles of the marathon!

Currently, no self-respecting coach, trainer, or athletic governing body would sanction such a primitive and physically dangerous policy. Most notably, this revised thinking about consuming fluids is underscored in virtually all training manuals. For example, virtually all cycling manuals now encourage riders to sip from their water bottles every 15 minutes — even when they don't feel thirsty. Failure to so, say the experts, could ultimately lead to dehydration.

While rehydration is no longer an issue, the same cannot be said for another time-honored sports tradition: the 'no pain, no gain' philosophy. Proponents of this crude concept believe that if athletes do not hurt while training, they stand little chance of making any progress.

Although the 'no pain, no gain' attitude has lost some ground, it continues to fight a rearguard action. That's because even the most enlightened athletes can be filled with doubt as to whether or not they are practicing hard enough.

Certainly no one would argue with the notion that hard work and dedication are two prerequisites for making advances in training and competition. But when elite and recreational athletes take this exercise tandem to the extreme, it frequently has dire consequences: *burn out* and overtraining, which can lead to a loss of enthusiasm for an activity, as well as illness and/or injury.

However, regardless of your level of ability, it is possible to avoid these pitfalls. To do so, you need an intelligently designed exercise program and remain sensitive to your mind and body. Furthermore, to reach the full potential in training and competition, it is essential to obtain objective, individualized information.

For today's athlete, one of the best means of acquiring this crucial data is by using a *heart rate monitor* (HRM). Although the HRM is a relatively new tool in the field of athletics, it has a long history in the medical profession. For decades, doctors

Fig. 0.1. Handlebar-mounted HRM with a sensor belt that can be worn over light clothing. See Chapter 3 for evaluation and selection guidelines.

have used various types of HRMs to keep tabs on patients afflicted with cardiac disorders. And over the years, coronary illness has claimed the lives of countless Americans.

Consider this: In a single year, heart maladies kill far more Americans than all of the US soldiers who died in wars during the 20th century. "I don't think people appreciate the fact that more than 50 percent of the deaths in this country are still due to heart disease," asserts Dr. Howard E. Morgan, a former President of the American Heart Association. These grim statistics clearly demonstrate that the heart plays a vital role in maintaining your overall well-being.

By monitoring the heart rate, an athlete is provided with information that will improve the efficiency of his or her body. That's because in one sense, the heart, metaphorically speaking, functions like your car's tachometer. As you drive away from a green light, the tachometer registers the engine's increasing revolutions per minute. Similarly, when your body works harder during exercise, the heart reveals this effort through an increasing number of beats per minute. Moreover, just as a race car driver employs a tachometer to improve his machine's performance, you, too, can use your heart — in conjunction with a HRM — to gauge, as well as optimize your health and fitness.

A common fallacy held by both active and sedentary people is that good health and optimum fitness are synonymous. That is not correct. Your fitness is measured by the ability to perform a physical task — which can range from an hour of leisurely riding or walking to competing in the Tour de France or running a marathon. Conversely, good health has nothing to do with athletic ability. Rather, it's a state where all your bodily systems are functioning harmoniously.

It's not unusual, then, to find athletes who are very fit, yet in a poor state of health at the same time. An example of this condition is the cyclist who breezes through daily workouts and is still plagued by colds or nagging injuries. (This all too common circumstance is indicative of an imbalanced training program — which can be restored to equilibrium through the correct use of a HRM.)

Worse yet, has been the recent spate of world-class athletes who have succumbed to heart attacks. Their ranks include running guru Jim Fix, basketball sharpshooters Hank Gathers and Pete Maravich, as well as several European professional bicycle racers.

Invariably, such tragedies are so shocking that many people begin to reflect on the quality of their lives. But all too often the impact soon fades, and then it's back to business as usual: jobs and personal relationships that induce excessive stress; diets that don't provide adequate nourishment or foster overweight problems. Generally, people who remain on a course that diminishes their health believe a heart attack — or another type of physical problem — is something that happens to someone else.

As someone who is already physically active, you are already on the road to a healthy lifestyle. This book is geared to help you achieve this eminently worthwhile objective. Its central premise is quite simple: The heart rate monitor, which is both sophisticated and user-friendly, can be used effectively to improve your overall well-being. By virtue of its precision, it can maintain the all-important symmetry of your training program. So, whether you are a fitness enthusiast or a competitive athlete, a HRM can take you to higher levels of health and conditioning.

This book explains how to evaluate a HRM's strengths and weaknesses, how the various devices function, and which models are the most appropriate for either fitness or competition.

Most importantly, the book reveals how to accurately calculate your individual *heart rate target zone*. By exercising within this parameter, you can attain superior conditioning and reduce the chances of sustaining debilitating illnesses and/or injuries. However, should you experience either one of these problems, you will learn how to facilitate your rehabilitation. Morover, the book shows how to apply your target zone data to both aerobic and anaerobic workouts — the two necessary exercise activities required to maintain and balance your health and fitness.

While bicycle racing is certainly one athletic discipline where the heart rate monitor has been used quite effectively (and indeed most of the examples in this book are based on cycling), cyclists are not the only athletes who can profit from this book: You will be shown how the training and competitive principles related to the HRM can be utilized by runners and swimmers, as well as by triathletes and biathletes. Given that the most modern HRMs are both reliable and affordable, it's the wise athlete who incorporates this device into his or her training program. Ultimately, this technology can provide a physiological window that will enable you to evaluate, control and promote your health and conditioning.

CHAPTER 1

A Matter of Balance: Aerobic and Anaerobic

While most athletes toss around the words *aerobic* and *anaerobic* as casually as their bike, swimming goggles or running shoes, they usually don't understand what these terms really mean. They commonly say aerobic means using oxygen, or the breathing pattern that accompanies long, steady exercising. Anaerobic is described as a state lacking oxygen — such as when ascending a steep hill, where breathing becomes extremely difficult.

These pedestrian definitions, which are neither accurate nor precise, were originated, in part, by microbiologists. Since some laboratory microbes required oxygen to live, researchers classified them as *aerobic*. Those microbes that couldn't survive in oxygen were, therefore, designated *anaerobic*.

Both of these nomenclatures are fine for microbes, but they hardly apply to people who run, swim or ride bicycles. Obviously, oxygen is essential for all of life's activities. Yet even the most well-conditioned athlete would be hard pressed to remain in a state void of oxygen for much more than a couple of minutes. In regard to aerobic and anaerobic, then, laboratory definitions definitely don't apply to human beings.

For the athlete, useful explanations of these two exercise patterns are instructive as well as significant. The most obvious distinction between aerobic and anaerobic activity is the different kind of fuel they rely on. Aerobic workouts, for the most part, utilize fat (fatty acids) as a source of energy, while anaerobic efforts are fueled by sugar (glucose). Consequently, the most practical meaning of each term is this: aerobic is the chemical state when the body is burning fat and anaerobic is the state when it burns sugar.

It is important to note that when you are burning sugar, you are not burning fat — and, frequently, your body is storing this substance.

Generally, the aerobic process, which relies on slow-twitch muscle fibers, contributes to your good health. It improves the heart's condition as well as blood circulation; it helps the body regulate fats and the hormonal system, and it enhances physical endurance. The anaerobic process cannot provide you with any of these benefits. That's because it is usually a product of intense exertion or competition which primarily involves an athlete's fast-twitch muscle fibers.

The obvious question, then, is how do you determine whether your workouts are aerobic or anaerobic? Simple: check your pulse with a HRM. Fluctuations in an athlete's heart rate occur simultaneously with changes in other bodily functions. As the pulse rate rises during a workout, there is a parallel increase in oxygen up-take (the amount of O_2 utilized), the rate of breathing, lactic acid, or blood lactate build-up.

While you are pedaling your bike or running at a comfortable aerobic pace, for example, your heart rate will probably remain at a relatively low level. In this easy exercise mode, the body derives most of its energy from fat. But later in the workout, you may start to really hammer. As your cadence gets progressively faster, your heart rate begins to rise and, as a result, more and more fuel is required. When the body reaches a point where it can no longer obtain energy from fat, it shifts to sugar for its fuel source. (The body converts sugar faster than fat into energy.) Beyond this point, the body is functioning anaerobically.

It is especially difficult for most athletes — regardless of their sport — to recognize when they have turned anaerobic. And after they have made this transition, it's not easy for them to get back into the aerobic state again. That's because the increase in lactic acid associated with anaerobic activity tends to suppress the body's aerobic functioning. So once you have become even mildly anaerobic, you will obtain considerably fewer aerobic benefits.

Consequently, you should not overlook the fact that, depending on your workout regimen, you are *training* the body to become either predominantly anaerobic or aerobic. Indeed,

Fig. 1.1. Nelson Vails' specialty is the short sprint race, essentially all anaerobic. In preparation and training for this kind of event, the heart rate monitor should play an important role. But this is one discipline in which the heart rate monitor is generally not used during the actual event.

this conditioning impression molded during exercise, continues, through a complex biochemical process, for as long as 48 hours after exercise.

Given all of the above information, it's a good bet that athletes who are continually in the throes of illness and/or injury are spending too much time working out anaerobically.

To achieve the necessary balance between the aerobic (fat-burning) and anaerobic (sugar-burning) states, it's essential to employ a HRM. But, in order to utilize this exercise device correctly, you must first establish your personal heart rate level. This critical information can literally be a lifesaver.

CHAPTER 2

Determining Your Heart Rate

Some well-heeled athletes who want to fine-tune their training and uncover secrets about their bodies' limits, spend quite a bit of time and money at sports physiology laboratories. There, health professionals put them through a rigorous battery of tests.

This research provides the athlete with a knowledge about his or her blood lactate and muscle lactic acid levels, maximum oxygen uptake, respiratory quotient, and heart rate. The last two factors are particularly valuable.

Respiratory quotient indicates how the body is utilizing oxygen and carbon dioxide. Through this assessment, it can be ascertained whether an athlete is primarily burning fat or sugar while exercising. This procedure is performed by measuring the amount of oxygen the body consumes and comparing it to the quantity of carbon dioxide exhaled. The mathematical ratio of carbon dioxide to oxygen is called RQ (Respiratory Quotient), or R Value. It ranges from 0.7 to 1.0. As an athlete's R Value gets closer to 0.7, it denotes that more fat is being used to fuel the body. And when the value tilts closer to 1.0, this suggests that sugar, in increasing amounts, is the dominant energy source.

The second factor — heart rate — can be used alone to conduct all the previously mentioned research that a sports lab performs. This is possible since the heart rate accurately parallels these other factors. In effect, there is an inexpensive and practical method for evaluating your physical condition as well as the effectiveness of your workouts right at your fingertips.

This was not always the case. Up until the last decade, there were only two heart rate evaluation procedures available: the *talk test* — which originated with the 1970's running craze — and a quasi-scientific formula based on an athlete's chronological age. When applying the talk test, it is assumed you are exercising within the aerobic range if you can *comfortably talk* to your training partners during a workout. This test, however, is about as reliable as the flip of a coin, since the chances are 50–50 you will be either right or wrong.

Given these odds, the quasi-scientific method seems infinitely more reliable for structuring a training program based on the athlete's heart rate. This system, which is widely used today, instructs riders to subtract their age from 220 and multiply the difference by a figure ranging from 65 to 85 percent. Supposedly, the resulting number provides the ath-

Fig. 2.1. The formulas in this chapter will help you establish your target heart rate curve much more accurately than by using the generalized target zone chart seen in many gyms and fitness studios.

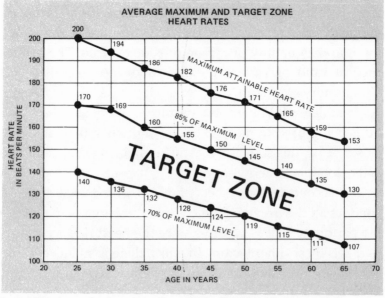

lete with the maximum heart beats per minute (bpm) for keeping workouts aerobic — or, rather, just at the *anaerobic threshold* (AT).

Technically, exercising at AT means you have reached the highest level of oxygen uptake, or the point at which, regardless of the workload, you can't consume any more oxygen. Yet, the term *threshold,* as defined in the AT method, refers to the onset of anaerobic exercise. This approach to training, therefore, emphasizes anaerobic efforts — however mild they may be — as opposed to aerobic activities.

The assumed rationale for this approach contains two fallacies. First, it assumes that 220 minus age will render an athlete's maximum pulse rate. But if you are to derive conditioning benefits by means of this equation you must push

---

Case History: Jack's Fatigue

Jack, a 38-year old businessman, had been riding his bike for 4 years to stay in shape. He began finding it impossible to train more than four days a week without taking a day or two off due to fatigue. Also, during the evenings after a ride, he would fall asleep early and had difficulty getting out of bed the next morning.

When Jack began working out with a HRM, he immediately disovered that his pulse rate rose above 170 bpm when climbing hills. This reading, as a consequence of his age, indicated he was definitely in an anaerobic state.

By using a HRM on all of his rides, Jack learned to climb bills at a pace dictated by his body. After about two weeks of training in the target zone, his pace on the hills began increasing, his energy returned, and he no longer felt compelled to go to bed early.

yourself to the max to make this formula work — otherwise it simply isn't valid. Second, the multiplier (65%–85%) is an arbitrary figure that doesn't consider an athlete's overall health and fitness.

Yet before dismissing this method, it's essential to examine the concept of AT-training. The leading exponent of this practice is the Italian physiologist Dr. Francesco Conconi. He was among the first in the sports medicine profession to bring his laboratory out on the road in order to work with cyclists. Conconi's pioneering efforts received widespread attention on January 23, 1984, due to the astounding achievement of the then 32 year old Italian racer Francesco Moser. Moser, who was trained by Conconi, established a new hour speed record for the bicycle — 51.151 km. Moser's accomplishment, especially in light of his age, sold the bicycling community an AT training.

Indeed, Conconi's AT concept was a real breakthrough as a way of training cyclists and other athletes.* In fact, some of the procedures outlined in this book parallel his work. The major differences between the information presented here and that offered by Conconi are in the realms of philosophy and physiology, as well as experience.

Conconi believes the ideal training level is achieved by exercising at your AT. *The High Performance Heart*, by contrast, takes the position that Maximum Aerobic Function (MAF) — the number of heart bpm that produces the most aerobic benefits with the least anaerobic stimulation — is the optimal

---

* Because the physiological basis of AT training is extremely complex, those desiring more detailed information on this subject should consult the study "Determination of the anaerobic threshold by a non-evasive field test in runners," by Conconi et al, published by the American Physiological Society in 1982.

method of obtaining fitness. That's because, as previously mentioned, the conditioning effect on your aerobic system is inhibited when you become even slightly anaerobic .

Athletes who utilize MAF-training, as opposed to AT-training, can be assured of several positive results: They will not only develop their anaerobic system — which is mandatory for competition — but they will also be moving in a direction that promotes good health. And to pursue a training program that may leave you fit but unhealthy makes little sense.

An accurate method to determine your heart rate is, therefore, essential for realizing your overall well-being. In a medical setting, ascertaining the exact relationship between heart rate and aerobic state is achieved by clinically establishing an athlete's *true*, or physiological, age. Different doctors do this in different ways. What they commonly evaluate, however,

---

Case History: Susan's Injuries

Susan, 29, was a cycling veteran of 10 years whose specialty was century rides. Still, she was continually plagued by injuries. When asked if she had ever ridden with a HRM, Susan replied, "Oh, I use one all the time." What she didn't use, however, was the proper formula to determine her target zone's parameters. Given Susan's age and the fact that she was experiencing health problems, her maximum training heart rate should have been around 146 bpm. Instead, she had calculated her top end at 155 bpm, believing that cycling experience was the most important factor.

Upon correctly using the 180 formula, Susan resumed her long distance cycling regimen — and was no longer beset by the persistent injuries.

---

are the lungs' vital capacity, blood sugar, and the condition of the heart (by using an electrocardiogram), as well as an individual's personal and family history.

What becomes readily apparent from such medical analysis is that a 40-year old athlete may have the body efficiency (the ability to perform an athletic task) of an individual either 10 years older or 20 years younger. (Kent Bostick, who helped power his squad to the 1990 United States National team time trial championship at age 37, clearly falls into the latter category.) As a consequence of physiological condition, the *true* age of these 40-year old athletes would be closer to 50 and 20, respectively.

Doctors can help athletes establish their correct heart rate. Yet it is quite possible to make this determination on your own with reasonable accuracy. All you have to do is to follow this easy 2-step formula:

Step 1:
Subtract your chronological age from 180.

Step 2:
Place yourself in one of the four categories below and adjust the number derived in Step 1 accordingly:

☐ If you have never trained before, are recovering from a major injury, operation, and/or illness, or are taking medication, subtract 10 from the number obtained in Step 1.

☐ If you are currently exercising, but have been falling short of your goals (e.g. improved fitness, better competitive results, more energy, weight loss, etc.), or your workout routine is inconsistent, or you have suffered an injury (even a minor one), or you have had more than 2 colds or cases of the flu during the past year, subtract 5 from the number obtained in Step 1.

☐ If for the past year you have worked out consistently (4 or more times per week), have progressed to your satisfaction (feel fitter, enjoyed improved competitive results, have more energy, lost weight, etc.) and have not suffered any injury or experienced no more than 2 colds or cases of the flu, do not alter the number obtained in Step 1.

☐ If you compete, and your performance has improved over the past two years, you have not suffered any injuries or experienced more than 2 colds or cases of the flu during the past year, then add 5 to the number obtained in Step 1.

More than likely, you will easily be able to find a suitable category and obtain a specific numerical value. This figure, regardless of the category, is the maximum heart rate that will keep you aerobic when training.

'In Between' Status

Some athletes, however, may be in a quandary over how to determine their exact maximum heart rate figure. That's because, due to a variety of circumstances, they feel as though they fall in between categories. If you are in this situation, just select the more conservative number.

Here is a typical example of an athlete who qualifies for 'in between' status. He is 35 years old and has been working out for 3 years — despite experiencing a nagging injury (e.g. a minor knee problem or lower back pain). If your situation is similar, no matter how old you are, compute your maximum heart rate in this manner:

Step 1:
180 minus age
$180 - 35 = 145$

Step 2:
Choose category b and subtract 5:
145 − 5 = 140

In this case, your maximum heart rate, therefore, would be 140 bpm. Generally, the figure derived this way will enable training without harming the body and still provide fat-burning, aerobic benefits. Should your heart rate exceed 140 bpm, however, you would not only start burning sugar, but also risk the possibility of aggravating the injury.

All athletes, upon arriving at a number that indicates their peak heart rate, should establish a *bpm range*. The most serviceable span is 10 bpm below your top-end, since it's often difficult to keep your heart rate at its designated maximum. If your maximum aerobic heart rate is 165 bpm, for example, you will still derive conditioning and health gains at your low-end of 155 bpm.

Since the 180-formula takes into account an athlete's health, as well as fitness, it will be more precise than its 220-counterpart. The 4 categories, however, are similar in rationale to the 65 to 85 percent multipliers prescribed in the 220-procedure. Yet, even in this area, the 180-method has demonstrated greater accuracy.

For the past decade, the 180-system has been used to clinically monitor the heart rates of athletes whose abilities ranged from superstar to novice. Morover, during this period, the 4-category plan has proven to be much more reliable than the percentage multiplier approach as a means of establishing an individual's maximum heart rate.

While the 180-equation can confirm your correct target zone, it does not guarantee your overall well-being. To reach a state where health and fitness are equally balanced, you must have a reliable means of recording your heart rate.

CHAPTER 3

Evaluating Heart Rate Monitors

Most athletes still rely on an antiquated, manual method for gauging their heart rate. During and after training, they place an index finger on the neck's carotid artery. Then they employ either the 6 or 10 second formula in hopes of determining their heart rate in bpm. (The former prescription calls for counting your heart rate for 6 seconds and multiplying by 10; the latter requires counting the beats for 10 seconds and multiplying by

Fig. 3.1. The heart rate monitor should always be worn directly around the chest wall cavity and never over clothing. Use water to moisten the electrode strap to improve contact with the skin. Since perspiration build-up hampers accurate recording of the heart rate, the strap should be periodically cleaned in a mild soapy water solution

29

6.) Certainly, this procedure is quite simple, but as for being accurate, that's an entirely different matter.

In order to take your pulse rate by hand, you must at least slow down. If nothing else, the termination or reduction of your workout pace means you are not measuring the *working* heart rate. As a result of this circumstance, the figure produced by both the 6 and 10-second methods can be off by as much as 10 to 15 bpm.

There are several common scenarios guaranteed to create unreliable manual heart rate readings. In the case of cycling, these include hill climbs and sprinting as well as performing speed work and intervals.

Let's take, for example, climbing a hill on a hot summer day. So, there you are, when it's 90 degrees in the shade, having just crested the summit of a tough ascent. Sweat is stinging your eyes, your quads are burning, and your mouth

Fig. 3.2. Many HRM's for use on stationary bikes have sensors that are clipped to the earlobe. However, at higher than moderate heart rates, these units become less accurate due to distortions in the pulses in the ear lobe.

is as dry as the Sahara Desert. You reach for your neck, attempting to gauge your rapidly thumping pulse. Good luck.

Here's another illustration depicting the obstacles cyclists must overcome when taking their heart rates manually. Imagine doing intervals in early November with the mercury hovering around 40°F (4°C). After each 100 meter dash, you feather the brakes and sit up — as a smokey, dragon-like breath pours out of your nose and mouth. You pull off one of your thermal gloves and place a finger inside your jacket collar and under that turtleneck. Several more seconds pass before you finally locate the carotid artery. Again, you will need a lot of good fortune to obtain an accurate pulse rate reading. On account of the multiplier used, if you happen to add or miss

Fig. 3.3. The Polar Cyclo Vantage is based on the latest technology and is intended for serious cyclists. It combines heart rate monitoring with the functions of a cyclo computer, measuring speed, cadence, distance and elapsed time. In addition, it retains data in memory for 8 hours and includes Conconi test information.

just one or two heart beats while counting, you can end up with a plus or minus of 20 bpm!

Need further proof about the limits of manual pulse-taking? Clinical research is available: Both recreational and world-class cyclists and triathletes were asked to wear HRMs during their prescribed workouts. When simultaneously measuring heart rates taken by hand with those registered on the monitors, the former readings were consistently lower.

Clearly, if you want hassle-free, accurate pulse rate information, you should rely on a HRM. Currently, there are two types of HRMs available on the market: the wired digital pulse-point unit and the wired or wireless chest wall devices. Both types of instruments come in a wide variety of models.

The pulse-point unit, operating on the principle of photo-reflectance, depends on a photo-cell and a light source to record your heart rate. A sensor equipped with a surgical rubber gripper is fastened to either the fingertip or earlobe. The passage of blood through the vessels in both extremities blocks out the light with each pulse beat. The receiver's timer circuitry, which can be clipped on to a runner's singlet or a cyclist's jersey, converts this information into a displayed heart rate.

The primary virtue of a pulse-point HRM is price. It can be purchased for between $25 to $50. But bear in mind that you get just what you pay for.

The technological limitations of a pulse-point monitor are considerable. While this type of HRM is acceptable for indoor use, it doesn't work well outdoors where the light source is inconsistent. Also, frequently the unit doesn't allow you to program the upper and lower reaches of your target zone. Consequently, cyclists will frequently have to take their eyes off the road — certainly not a safe practice — to see their heart rate on the receiver. Furthermore, this device is extremely sensitive to body movements, so its accuracy becomes questionable during intense exertion — such as when thrusting a bike from side to side during a demanding hill climb.

Despite these constraints, the pulse-point device is definitely more accurate than manual pulse taking and the talk test. Yet this type of HRM will prove unsatisfactory if you are seriously concerned about fitness and/or competition.

In order to get the most out of your workouts, at least invest in a wired chest wall HRM. This instrument is much more accurate than its pulse-point counterpart, because it reads the heart's electrical activity. These electrical impulses, which are transmitted through the skin, are picked up by a comfortable lightweight chest belt equipped with rubber-covered sensors. The heart rate data is transmitted by a wire (which can be routed through the sleeve of your jersey) to the wristwatch-

Fig. 3.4. The Polar Optimex is for use on a stationary bike. The transmitter is worn around the chest and the receiver is mounted on the bike. It provides information about your high and low aerobic ranges, measures total elapsed time and stores information on exercise time spent in your target zone.

like receiver. If a cyclist chooses to mount the receiver on the handlebars, the wire can be run out the jersey's bottom or collar and secured to the frame's top tube.

The more sophisticated units offer a feature that is essential for all athletes, regardless of their exercise regimen: audible upper and lower alarm signal settings that can he precisely pre-programmed to the target zone. When you hear the alarm beeping, you know it's time to increase or decrease your effort.

The wired HRM has some drawbacks, however. The cable joining the chest belt's sensors to the receiver can restrict your movements, and it may be inadvertently disconnected or become entangled — which could cause a severe accident on a bicycle. These disconcerting qualities notwithstanding, expect to pay between $100–$175 for this type of unit.

The best all-around HRM is the wireless chest wall telemetry instrument. Cordless, it relies on radio waves to trans-

Fig. 3.5. With a computer, you can plot out your progress for a truly scientific approach to training. With the appropriate hardware and software, you can keep track of your workouts. Examples of such graphs are shown in Chapter 4.

mit your heart information from the chest strap sensors to its wristwatch-like receiver. Like the wired unit, the telemetric monitor has clock and stopwatch functions, as well as pre-programmable alarms to signal that you are exercising above or below the target zone. Like its cable correlate, the receiver can be mounted on a bike's handlebars. These features enable you to keep your eyes on the road, since you can either hear or momentarily glance at your heart rate quotient. Furthermore, because a telemetric HRM operates without wires, there's nothing to become entangled, disconnected, or to restrict your body's movements.

Other available options on some of these monitors include the ability to record the amount of time you have spent in the target zone, the displaying and cataloguing of split times, and the availability of cadence and altimeter functions. And swimmers will appreciate that some models are waterproof.

The top-of-the-line model has the capacity to store up to 8 hours of exercise statistics for as many as 15 races or workout sessions. Moreover, this performance information can be down-loaded to a personal computer. The interface package contains the necessary software to enable you to make an in-depth analysis of your heart rate data.

Because telemetric HRMs are precise and versatile, they are also very costly. Depending on the model you select, be prepared to fork out anywhere from $125 to $499.

Regardless of the HRM you choose — pulse-point, wired or wireless chest wall — your money will be well spent, because next to your bike, swimming suit or running shoes, it will be your most important piece of training equipment. Consider this: The heart rate monitor essentially provides you with the equivalent of a personal coach who gives you immediate feedback. And because the HRM is accurate and objective, it can effectively help you meet your goals for fitness or competition.

CHAPTER 4

Warming Up and Cooling Down: Keys to Health and Fitness

When asked to explain their warm-up and cool-down routines, many athletes express bewilderment or disdain. Others, who do take the time to perform these tasks, assume a very casual attitude. As for warming up, they say they spend a few minutes taking it easy before going all out. And their cool-down period concludes the moment they have caught their breath. If any of these responses reflect your opening and

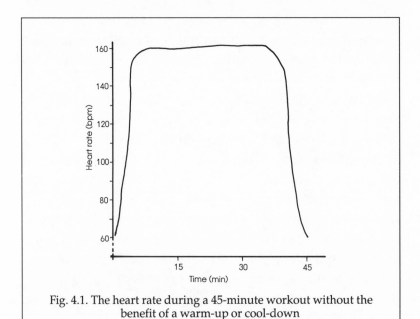

Fig. 4.1. The heart rate during a 45-minute workout without the benefit of a warm-up or cool-down

closing exercise patterns, you are a candidate for health and/or fitness problems.

Warming up and cooling down are the two most essential elements of any training program. Neglecting the former practice can cause overuse injuries, while ignoring the latter can diminish the gains derived from exercising. In terms of heart rate, this is the situation illustrated in Fig. 4.1.

The Warm-Up

When your body is at rest, most of the blood is circulating through the organs and glands — such as the adrenal and thyroid, the liver, kidneys, and pancreas — as well as other primary areas — like the nerves, brain, heart and intestines. How you treat these organs and glands at the onset — and at the conclusion — of a workout, effects not only your conditioning but also your overall health.

Fig. 4.2. The heart rate during a 60-minute workout. During the warm-up, the heart rate *slowly* rises to the maximum training level after about 15 minutes. The cool-down begins about 15 minutes before the end of the workout. During this period, the heart rate is slowly lowered, ending just above the starting heart rate.

As you first begin to exercise, your heart rate naturally increases, and more blood is *shunted* to the muscles engaged in the activity. As with any other sudden dramatic change to your body, the rapid redistribution of blood — away from the organs and glands, to the active muscles — can be very stressful. To ensure that you don't incur any physical damage, this blood redistribution process, or shunting, should occur very gradually. This gradual shunting of blood away from the organs and glands into the working muscles is the definition — as well as the purpose — of warming up.

Case History: Fred's Warm-Up

After several years of inactivity, 33-year old Fred was experiencing some difficulty motivating himself to get back into exercising. Finally, he took his old ten-speed out of the garage and began riding regularly again.

Even though Fred rode 5 days a week for three consecutive months, he felt he wasn't making any progress. Upon evaluating this situation, it was discovered that as soon as Fred rode away from the house, he began to climb a very steep hill. By having him use a HRM, he quickly noticed that after completing this ascent, his pulse rate had skied to 175 bpm. Once he descended and was on the flats, his heart rate came down to 140 bpm — which was appropriate for his age and level of fitness.

It was recommended that Fred warm-up thoroughly for 15 minutes and avoid climbing during this period. He took these suggestions and as a result saw a dramatic improvement in his overall performance.

A warm-up period at a low output level (i.e. using low gears in the case of cycling, a slow pace for runners and swimmers) for 10 to 15 minutes will allow your heart rate to rise gradually and prepare the body for the demands of exercising. The HRM plays a crucial role in this procedure. It keeps you aware of your pulse rate figures and their relationship to the shunting factor.

Figure 4.2 illustrates a proper warm-up with regard to heart rate and time for a one-hour aerobic workout, for an athlete whose maximum pulse is 145 bpm. In this example, the first 12 minutes are devoted to warming up. At the end of this time period, the heart rate should be in the target zone. Should a workout exceed 1½ hours, then the warm-up time should be extended to 20 minutes.

Figure 4.3 shows how an athlete who will be working out for 2 hours gradually and safely brings the heart rate into the target zone.

Fig. 4.3. During a longer workout of two hours, both the warm-up and the cool-down are expanded to about 30 minutes.

The Cool-Down

Equally significant as preparing your body for rigorous activity is giving it fair warning that the workout is ending. This is the cool-down period. If you don't take the time to perform this task correctly, too much blood tends to remain, or *pool*, in the muscles. When pooling occurs, the normal circulation of blood is impeded.

During the cool-down, the blood must be gradually recirculated back to the organs and glands. In the immediate post-exercise phase, blood is used for oxygen and nutrients necessary to repair the cells that were engaged during training or competition. Also the removal of waste — such as cellular debris and carbon dioxide — generated during activity is dependent upon good circulation. Consequently, if you don't take the time to cool-down adequately, blood pools in the muscles and reduces some of the health benefits of exercising.

The duration of the cool-down segment should correspond proportionally to the time you have been working out.

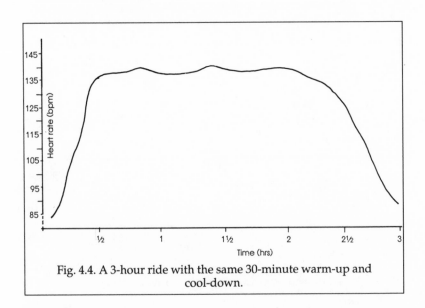

Fig. 4.4. A 3-hour ride with the same 30-minute warm-up and cool-down.

Figure 4.4 illustrates an athlete involved in a 3-hour practice session. This individual's maximum pulse rate is 165 bpm. Twenty to 30 minutes are spent warming up and 20 to 30 minutes will be spent cooling down.

The Warm-Up and Cool-Down Tandem: Some Special — and Not So Special — Circumstances

Let's assume you are pressed for time and can only exercise for half an hour; or that you're a novice and this is the extent of your training program. In either one of these instances, you will spend most of your exercise time just warming up and cooling down. And even when this is the length of your training session, you can still accumulate fitness assets.

Figure 4.5 illustrates an athlete whose pulse rate should not exceed 135 bpm, exercising for 30 minutes. In this case, the warm-up and the cool-down periods are 15 minutes each.

More than likely, this illustration provokes the question how only warming up and cooling down can provide any

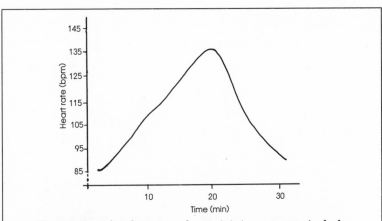

Fig. 4.5. Even for shorter workouts, it is important to include 12–15-minute warm-up and cool-downs. In this instance, the maximum heart rate is not maintained for long at all. This workout is mostly warming up and cooling down, but still provides many health benefits.

fitness and/or health benefits. Exercise can be defined in numerous ways. One definition is that it's the increase in the body's metabolism, or metabolic rate, beyond a resting state. What is really significant, then, is how much time is required to make this transition.

Most athletes, whether they are fit or out of shape, can make this shift in about 12 minutes. Consequently, they not only have enough time to warm up and cool down, but also briefly work in the target zone. An individual who regularly spends 10 or more hours per week exercising should not scoff at the value of occasional 30-minute sessions. Indeed, over the long haul, these short journeys will definitely be a boon to both health and conditioning.

Figure 4.6 represents an athlete training for 45 minutes. Observe that the only major difference between this and the previous example is the amount of time — 15 minutes — spent maintaining the maximum heart rate of 135 bpm.

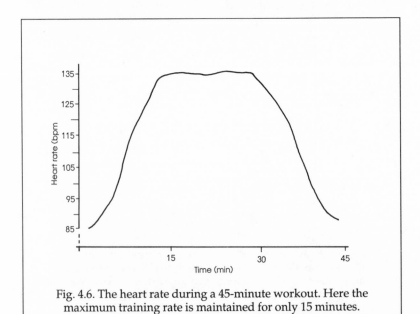

Fig. 4.6. The heart rate during a 45-minute workout. Here the maximum training rate is maintained for only 15 minutes.

Since people in general, and athletes in particular, tend to compare themselves with one another, note this well: The heart rates of two athletes can be radically different, even when they are both performing at the same output level. This can — and will — happen due to the differences in individuals' unique physical ability and body chemistry. So, even if you are a cyclist who can keep up with Tour de France winner Greg LeMond, don't expect to have the same heart rate as he does.

Ultimately, the best reason to warm up and cool down adequately is that both of these tasks can greatly reduce your

---

Case History: Jonathan's Tension

When cycling, 48-year old Jonathan took extreme care to keep his heart rate within the correct target zone. Since his body was often tight upon getting out of bed, he wisely spent at least 15 minutes warming up on early morning training rides. But Jonathan had a hectic daily schedule crammed with family, business, and social responsibilities. Therefore, to save a few minutes, he would come racing into his driveway at the and of a ride.

Sometimes, within an hour after a workout, his muscles would cramp and stiffen up. When this happened, he gobbled down two aspirins to ease the stress on his body. 'I just don't have the time,' Jonathan said, after being told he needed to spend 15 minutes cooling down. Yet he agreed to follow this procedure for one week, and was amazed that such a seemingly little thing could make such a big difference in how he felt. Free of the post-ride aspirin, Jonathan feels good all day, and his morning tightness has begun to dissipate.

chances of sustaining an injury. Studies show that athletes who don't engage in these routines are more prone to physical problems than those who scrupulously perform these activities.

For both the casual exerciser and world-class athlete, a HRM removes the guesswork from the warming up and cooling down periods. Don't dismiss the value of these pre- and post-workout functions just because you're not pushing your body to its maximum. Take the time to get up to and down from speed gradually. This will ensure that you get the most out of your training program.

CHAPTER 5

Training With a Heart Rate Monitor

Most athletes — especially those interested in competition — can benefit from a yearly training program. Each day can be put to good use, whether it's devoted to working out, racing, recovering, or simply maintaining your equipment. But even if you're not interested in competition, a 12-month training schedule is still very valuable. Besides giving your workouts a daily, as well as a long-range focus, it enables you to follow two critical rules while exercising:

Rule Number 1:
All of your aerobic workouts should be performed in the target zone. Even though your emphasis is on Maximum Aerobic Function, it's quite possible to become 'too aerobic.' In order to maintain a balance in your physical conditioning, there are times throughout the year that you must engage in anaerobic activities. Using a HRM for this type of exercise — whether it be sprints, intervals, and/or racing — is very important, since it allows you to safely push your body to the prescribed threshold.

Rule Number 2:
In order to objectively evaluate your physical conditioning, it is necessary to establish several performance benchmarks. By doing this, you can regularly note any changes in fitness. For example, by comparing the weekly times it takes to ride the same 10-mile loop in the target zone, you will obtain concrete knowledge as to whether or not you're making fitness advan-

ces. Furthermore, at the conclusion of every workout, you should become aware of another crucial conditioning reference point — recovery time, or how long it takes the heart rate to return to 'normal' after the stress of exercising.

Athletes intent on improving their health and fitness must adhere to these fundamental training axioms. And due to its aforementioned virtues, a HRM is an indispensable tool for maintaining these exercise principles.

Before designing your yearly training program, it's advisable to take 6 factors into consideration:

1. Scheduling:

Very few of us are going to become world-class athletes. Keeping this in mind, be realistic when creating your exercise calendar. Make sure you leave enough time to fulfill your responsibilities to family and friends, comfortably meet your work and/or education commitments, and still have the op-

Fig. 5.1 and Fig. 5.2. In addition to developing line graphs of your workouts, the computerized heart rate programs allow you to shift to bar charts (below) and numerical charts (facing page). The program also has a built-in Conconi calculation to determine your anaerobic threshold.

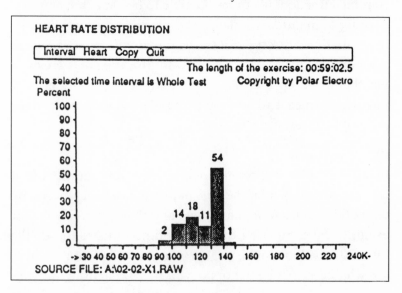

portunity for leisure activities. By taking all of these factors into account, you will have a better chance of sticking to your training schedule and, therefore, successfully integrating exercise into your lifestyle.

2. Physical Condition:

Ask yourself this basic question: Am I able to withstand the stress of daily exercising? If you have any uncertainty about your response, see a sports doctor and get a thorough physical check-up.

3. Biochemical Issues:

Because you are about to make some considerable demands on your body, it's important to provide it with the proper nutrients. Eating foods with fats will be necessary in order to attain aerobic efficiency. People with a penchant for eating sweets should note that sugary snacks and drinks tend to suppress the aerobic system. Therefore, If you feel compelled to fulfill this craving, don't do it just before exercising.

HEART RATE LISTING

NextPage	PreviousPage	Hardcopy	Interm.	Next	Quit

Copyright by POLAR ELECTRO   SOURCE FILE: Noname

Time   Heart Rate Values

Time											
00:00	78	77	76	73	73	74	77	81	82	78	74	74
00:01	76	76	76	75	78	76	75	75	75	76	77	76
00:02	77	77	76	80	87	88	81	76	72	75	77	75
00:03	75	75	79	80	77	82	79	73	74	75	76	73
00:04	70	73	77	81	79	80	79	78	74	77	75	73
00:05	71	69	70	72	72	75	75	81	78	75	73	73
00:06	71	72	75	74	77	77	73	75	75	78	80	77
00:07	77	73	73	71	71	68	71	77	73	79	83	83
00:08	82	84	83	81	78	0	77	69	71	74	74	72
00:09	73	78	75	72	74	79	75	75	76	75	73	68

Final Time: 00.05.28

Intermediate Times:

HR 103   HR 166   HR 113
00.01.48,6   00.38.30,7   00.05.26,5

HR 170   HR 179
00.26.02,3   00.41.25,2

---

4. Psychological Issues:
Studies have shown that when people exercise in the morning, as opposed to the evening, they have a greater chance of staying with a regular training program. Yet, whether you choose to train in the morning or the afternoon, adhere to a consistent schedule. Knowing *when* you are supposed to ride will encourage the maintenance of your routine. (All of this is not to say that some athletes don't possess the discipline to train at different times on different days, should they want to.)

For the purpose of organization, self-analysis, and motivation, keep a training diary. Each day, enter the following data: your morning pulse — which should be taken before getting out of bed — how long you remained in the target during your workout, and a few words about what you did, or did not, accomplish.

Regardless of whether you are exercising for fitness or competition, be realistic about the goals you are setting. Unless you are extremely talented, don't expect to establish any long distance records or win a lot of races during your first year of training or competition. Some people who set unrealistic goals become discouraged and give up if they find out they can't fulfill their unrealistic expectations. That's the last thing you want to happen.

Tailor your goals to your age and ability. In the case of cycling, some reasonable objectives may include riding continuously for 60 minutes, completing a fifty mile ride, or finishing with the pack during a race. No matter where you're positioned on the exercise spectrum, there is a value to reflecting on your goals and developing the correct strategy to meet them.

5. Habit Changes:
Sedentary individuals choosing to launch a training program are, first of all, changing their habits. And altering a deep-

seated habit is extremely difficult. For some people, just allotting time in the day to exercise can be a more formidable task than the workout itself.

When you begin a workout regimen, you may be cultivating a new mind-set; consequently it may be useful to adopt the notion that you are in the process of creating a positive addiction. In effect, you will be repeating an activity on a daily basis that will both nourish and excite your mind and body. How long it takes to develop this exercise pattern, and its associated responses, depends on your degree of commitment.

Generally, many novice athletes see their commitment begin to waver at two very specific moments. Initially, they have trouble mustering the requisite energy that will take them from the easy chair to their bicycle or other exercise equipment. Once they have surmounted that obstacle, inevitably,

Fig. 5.3. Heart rate monitor software will plot your workout with great accuracy. This 40 km time trial shows a fairly consistent racing heart rate throughout.

49

they face another rough spot: At some point during the first month of training, they will experience a loss of enthusiasm.

Being aware of such snares has some value. However, an effective way of avoiding both of these unsettling circumstances is to make plans to join forces with people who have already established a training routine. If you opt for this kind of psychological support from experienced friends, don't make the mistake of trying to keep pace with them. This could prove extremely discouraging. Instead, go at your own speed and make plans to meet them at designated points.

6. Time:

For both novice and seasoned athletes, most workouts should be based on time, rather than miles or laps. Time is a qualitative factor. And the body responds much better to the stress of time than the stress of distance, which is decidedly quantitative.

With regard to the issue of time, neophytes would profit from adopting the attitude that less is more. Why? Short exercise sessions reduce your chances of sustaining an injury; help keep your enthusiasm at a high level; and, most importantly, fosters the exercise habit. Given all of these factors, those who are just beginning an exercise regimen should not work out any longer than 30 minutes per session during the first 2 to 3 months.

However, certainly in the case of cycling, extended workout periods, as well as longer distances, do assume significance for experienced athletes. Both of these elements have to be taken into consideration, for example, when performing long, steady rides, speed work, and intervals. In such instances, numbers (miles, time, and heart rate) allow cyclists to adapt their training program to how they feel (rested or tired) and prepare for competition.

After you have taken all of these six factors into consideration, you are ready to formulate a personal yearly training program. A sample is listed below for a cyclist, while this regimen can be adapted easily for other forms of exercise.

Yearly Training Program for Competitive and Non-Competitive Cyclists

☐ November 15 to December 1: Rest Period

☐ December 1 to April 1: Aerobic Base and Cross-Training

☐ April 1 to July 1: Incorporate Anaerobic Training and Racing

☐ July 1 to August 15: Aerobic Base and Break from Racing

☐ August 15 to November 15: Incorporate Anaerobic Training and Racing

This 365-day schedule allows both competitive and non-competitive athletes ample time to develop their aerobic and anaerobic systems. The program's key feature, which will enable you to reach this two-fold objective, is, in a word, *specificity*. That means at various times of the year, you will be working on particular aspects of your health and/or conditioning. In order to truly harmonize both of these dimensions, it is crucial to be ruthlessly objective. And when it comes to presenting impartial, precise information about your body, there's no better device than a HRM.

Rest Period (November 15 to December 1)

Most likely, you will welcome the onset of these two weeks. It's free time to do whatever you like. And, most importantly, the Rest Period provides a psychological break from your workout regimen. But remember, just because you are on a vacation from training, doesn't mean you should overeat, drink to excess, and totally ignore your body. Use these two weeks wisely: Besides resting and relaxing, take some fun rides or participate in some non-demanding sports activity. To do otherwise may cause you to pay the piper during the next phase of your training program.

Aerobic Base and Cross-Training (December 1 to April 1)

Having rejuvenated your mind and body, you're probably more than ready to begin training in earnest. Your reintroduction to serious exercise begins with developing your aerobic base. Put simply, this is the period of time in the yearly training plan when you should engage only in aerobic activity. Consequently, you will not perform any anaerobic workouts — and that means not competing in other sports disciplines, such as

Fig. 5.4. When viewed after training, certain inconsistencies, such as the cadence in this 2 hr 15 min workout, become apparent.

track and cyclocross races, cross-country skiing, swimming, and running competitions, etc. unless, of course, you can remain in the aerobic range.

Rebuilding the aerobic system correctly requires several months of abstaining from anaerobic activity. That's because anaerobic exercise can interfere with aerobic progress, or your ability to do more work at any given heart rate.

Depending on the individual, and his or her level of fitness, anaerobic workouts can produce varied consequences. For the extremely fit and healthy person, these intense efforts will usually cause only a mild disruption of aerobic progress. On the other hand, if you are not in great shape, or have been ill and/or injured, anaerobic workouts can bring about major training setbacks: You will either endure the termination of all aerobic benefits, and/or experience an actual regression in aerobic fitness.

The reason why anaerobic activity can hinder aerobic functioning is not entirely clear. One known connection, however, is that lactic acid — which is increasingly produced during anaerobic activity — can interfere with the body's chemical functions that enables aerobic metabolism to take place.

To ensure that aerobic metabolism takes place without any impediments, most athletes would, in fact, profit from bi-annual aerobic base periods. The longer rebuilding stage should begin in early December and last until mid-March, and a shorter, two-week, mid-summer term would start in early July and continue on into mid-August.

The time you will spend re-establishing your aerobic base is not written in stone. Typically, the first, and longer period lasts from two to four months. Some athletes, however, will require a greater or lesser duration to satisfy this essential fitness objective.

How long it takes to fully replenish the aerobic system depends on a variety of factors. If you have suffered bouts of illness and/or injuries, or have seen a steady decline in your performances, add one or two months to the regular aerobic base period. Conversely, if you are satisfied with both your race results and/or level of fitness, and you have remained healthy, your aerobic base period may be as brief as two months.

Cross-Training

While you are in the process of revitalizing your aerobic system, take the opportunity to participate in some cross-training. One of the problems of becoming a single-sport specialist is that you don't realize your full body potential.

Many cyclists who are in reasonably good shape, for example, are unable to run up a long flight of stairs without gasping for breath! When racers, in particular, experience this situation, they usually exclaim something like, 'I can't believe it! How could this happen?' Easy: It's the result of working out exclusively on their bicycles.

Generally, running — whether it's in the hills or on the flats — utilizes a set of muscle groups that the pedaling motion fails to develop. Moreover, when you sprint in sneakers, as opposed to sprinting on a bicycle, it makes different demands on your nervous system. And, if nothing else, cross-training's fundamental purpose is to educate your nervous system so that it can respond to a wide variety of exercises.

To reach this objective, cyclists can participate in any one of many activities during the aerobic base period. These include swimming, cross-country skiing, ice skating, rowing and even dancing and speed-walking. In many cases, cross-training may be a desirable alternative to cycling when the weather interferes with your activity on the bicycle.

Outdoor Riding in Cold Weather

If you live where the cold winds blow and the snow falls, it's imperative to take several precautions when riding outdoors. These warnings apply specifically to cycling, but to some extent may also be applicable when running.

☐ When the temperature drops below 50° Farenheit (10° C), be sure to wear the proper clothing. Even though this may seem obvious, many cyclists still fall victim to frostbite injuries. The best way to ward off extremely cold weather is to dress in heat-conserving layers, topped-off with wind-resistant thermals (jacket, tights, gloves, and booties). These garments are said to wick away moisture, but if you tend to sweat a lot, make sure the HRM is waterproof.

☐ Roads covered with snow and ice pose grave threats even to the most intrepid cyclists. Those riders driven to work out under these hazardous conditions should invest in a

Fig. 5.5. A steady heart rate is generally a sign of high efficiency during competition.

mountain bike. This low-to-the-ground machine, outfitted with road-gripping knobby tires, will give you a fighting chance to remain upright on slippery surfaces.

☐ Regardless of the bike you are riding or the clothes you are wearing, bear in mind that the wind chill factor can be devastating, cooling your body much more than the air temperature may suggest.

☐ Even outdoors in winter, all your workouts require warm-up and cool-down periods. Avoid the unhealthy tendencies to pedal faster at the onset of activity and to skip the cool-down period altogether. If the temperature is too low to perform these procedures, start and end your training session on a windload simulator or on rollers.

Windload Simulators

Many cyclists who want to remain fit throughout the winter commonly rely on a windload simulator, or turbo-trainer. The equipment is a breeze to use. All that's required is slipping-off the bike's front wheel (on some models even that is not necessary) and securing the fork into the trainer's quick-release assembly. The frame is mounted and clamped to the stand at its bottom bracket or held in place at the rear wheel axle. The rear wheel acts on a cylinder that drives wind turbines (or their inductive substitute). As you pedal and shift into higher gears, the resistance increases exponentially, similar to the wind resistance during outdoor cycling.

More often than not, cyclists become quite bored during windload simulator workouts. In an attempt to divert themselves while getting nowhere fast, they read, watch television, or listen to music. Yet this task can be made entertaining and instructive, as well as more productive, simply by using a cyclocomputer (a device that measures speed, distance, pedaling rate, etc) and a HRM.

While observing these instruments while riding a windload simulator, you will probably notice some significant changes in your efforts. More than likely, you will be able to ride harder and faster in your prescribed target zone, as compared to cycling outdoors. Let's assume, for example, that your average road speed is 15 miles per hour while you're in the target zone. On a windload simulator, however, you may be able to simulate a riding speed that is 2 or 3 miles per hour faster — without any alteration in your normal heart rate.

This increased speed at the same pulse rate is caused by two factors: a decrease in humidity and less resistance. The difference between your outdoor and indoor speeds will increase over time and will be quite a bit greater when you conclude this training at the end of the winter.

To verify this observation, use a cyclocomputer in conjunction with your HRM. Once a week, either perform a 1-hour or a 25 mile time trial or administer the Maximum Aerobic Function examination. (See in the section *Plotting Heart Rate, Speed or Distance, and Time: The MAF-Test.*)

A windload simulator provides cyclists with an opportunity to perform out-of-the-saddle sprints and speed-work, along with intervals. Limit all of these workout routines to 1 hour and 15 minutes — to ride longer usually promotes boredom and a lack of enthusiasm for this task. And, of course, never omit your warm-up and cool-down segments.

Rollers

Rollers, unlike windload simulators, are not equipped with a bicycle support system. Upon placing your bike upon the unit's three spinning drums, you have to balance it while you are pedaling, treadmill-fashion. Indeed, this approach to indoor training demands your complete attention. To do otherwise could send you tumbling into a piece of living room furniture.

Still, many cyclists are willing to take this inherent risk that comes with riding rollers. Along with keeping them focused, the apparatus definitely improves their form and pedaling technique, as well as their balance.

Adept roller riders can engage in the same indoor workouts as those who rely on windload simulators. Yet, due to the tension associated with trying to remain vertical, they may not experience a similar drop in their target zone pulse rate.

Plotting Heart Rate, Speed or Distance, and Time: The MAF-Test.

Sometime during the Aerobic Base Period, you will want to evaluate your fitness status. What guideline, then, is available to determine whether you are actually progressing or regressing, or on the verge of an injury and/or illness? The way to obtain all of this critical information is by measuring your Maximum Aerobic Function (MAF) with a HRM.

By comparing your heart rate with speed, distance, and/or time (if your HRM does not have the ability of recording all of these data, it will be necessary to also employ a cyclocomputer), you will know exactly where you stand.

If you live in a cold climate, you can administer the MAF-test while exercising indoors in winter. Then, when the weather becomes conducive to outdoor exercise, you will periodically do this test on your test course.

In cycling, the ideal place to conduct the MAF-test is a velodrome. But since these banked, oval tracks are few and far between, you will probably have to find a substitute. The next best location is a stretch of open road, preferably a loop that can be ridden continuously — i.e. it must be free from traffic lights and stop signs and other obstacles that would force you to slow down or stop riding.

In this reasonably safe zone, you can determine your MAF. First warm up for 15 minutes, making sure your heart rate reaches its target zone parameters. Having done this, ride your test course. Let's say that on your first effort you cover the circuit in 14 minutes. For the next 3 months, repeat the MAF-test once a week, making sure to record your times in your training diary after each effort.

If all goes well during these 12 weeks, you will probably build up your aerobic base. Your increasing fitness will be clearly indicated by the time reduction(s) on your test circuit.

One caveat: Time improvements in cycling are rarely constant or linear. Here's a typical bicycle scenario that exemplifies this phenomenon. Suppose after 3 months of consistent training, you have brought your test course time down from 14 to 12 minutes. Then, one day, you're suddenly jolted: It takes you 15 minutes to complete the circuit! Don't panic. There are several possible explanations for this apparent regression.

Often, the reason for a single increased test time is that you are simply having a bad day — and that even happens to top echelon racers. A bad day can be attributed to several factors, some of which may be signaled by higher morning heart rates. For instance, you may have a cold or the flu coming on. Then, too, you may be experiencing excessive stress at home, work, or school. Still another possibility is that you could be a little burned-out from overtraining.

Eventually, through self-analysis, you may be able to rectify some of these performance-detracting circumstances. Other factors, such as those listed below, however, will clearly be out of your control:

1. High humidity:

A cyclist will incur more riding resistance as the percentage of water in the air increases. As a result, it requires more effort to pedal a bike, which is evidenced by higher heart rates and increased MAF times.

2. Low Barometric Pressure.:

When the barometric pressure is falling, it reduces the body's ability to take up oxygen. This means you will have to expend more energy — as indicated by a rise in your heart rate — to achieve your usual results. A quick check of your local newspaper's weather map can tell you if this factor may be the reason for your weaker performance.

3. Wind resistance:

Cycling into a head wind requires a higher work output at the same speed, elevates the heart rate and can also lead to biochemical problems.

If, on the other hand, your test course times either plateau or improve only slightly, there is nothing to worry about. As your MAF functions develop — with months and years of training — your rate of progress will become more moderate.

Don't expect to see any radical improvements in your test times during the anaerobic and/or competitive segment of your yearly training plan. During those periods, you have amassed your maximum aerobic benefits. Yet, should your test course times become significantly slower in this phase, it's a good bet you are either overtrained (doing too many anaerobic workouts) or racing too frequently.

Recovery Time

The MAF-test offers both novice and elite athletes the opportunity to evaluate another component in the fitness equation:

recovery time, i.e. how long it takes the heart rate to return to normal after the stress of exercise. An effective training program should promote faster recovery time, regardless of the duration of your daily workout — it could be as short as 30 minutes or as long as 1½ hours.

Most cyclists are interested in getting in their miles. Yet, sometimes, that one workout, whether 5 miles or 50, could leave you overtrained if your body has not adequately recovered from earlier exertions. This athletic malady, *overtraining*, can easily be avoided by using the HRM in conjunction with the following guidelines:

☐ Make sure that you are aware of your initial heart rate before every workout.

☐ At the conclusion of each training session, adhere to the cool-down procedure as explained in Chapter 4. This ensures that your body will sufficiently recover from the effort of training.

☐ Observe your heart rate during the cool-down period. More than likely, the number of bpm will not have returned to the pre-exercise level. This is to be expected and indicates that you require more time to achieve full recovery.

Depending on your physical condition, it may take between 1 and 2 hours for your heart rate to get back to normal. And if you are new to the sport, your recovery may require an even longer term. If you are extremely fit, on the other hand, your pulse rate may drop down to its pre-exercise level within minutes. Bear in mind that the intensity of a ride does effect recovery time. An hour's hammering uphill, for instance, requires a longer recovery time than the same time spent on a slow, steady ride.

☐ Continue to wear the HRM for a couple of hours after your ride (this will require briefly removing the device while you're in the shower, unless you have a waterproof model). As you go through your post-exercise routine, you will probably find that your heart rate fluctuates slightly.

After a month or two of monitoring yourself in this fashion, you will have a good idea how long it takes you to recover from different types of exercise activities. With increasing fitness, your post-exercise pulse rate should move closer and closer to the pre-exercise level — so long as you don't suffer any physical problems.

Some athletes, however, may discover that their heart rate is not decreasing during the post-exercise period. There is nothing to worry about if that happens. Generally, it implies that the exercise was simply too stressful. Assuming this is the case, it will be reflected the next day by a higher than normal morning pulse rate, as discussed in the next chapter. If you find yourself in this situation, simply comply with the following prescription: Keep your heart rate at the lower end of the target zone on your next ride.

☐ When performing intervals and speed work, make sure that your heart rate drops down below your aerobic range after each hard effort. Let's say your target zone is 150–160 bpm, and the interval brings your heart rate up to 180 bpm. Don't engage in another interval until you see that your heart rate has settled back into the high 140's.

☐ Racers should follow the same basic recovery procedures as mentioned above. However, due to the physical demands of competition, their recovery times are usually longer. Often, the heart rates of cyclists who have participated in a race do not return to the pre-competition level for several hours — or even several days.

If you are a racer and your pulse rate remains above normal for more than a day or two, it may indicate one, or all, of the following problems: your racing form was inadequate (specifically, a greater aerobic base was required); the race was physically too demanding and, as a result, it may eventually cause an illness and/or an injury; or the recovery was incomplete for reasons that may include an injury, dehydration, or a nutritional deficiency.

☐ Wear your HRM for an entire day. When you are not exercising, turn the target zone signals off and regularly glance at the display. Using your morning pulse rate as the base figure, you can learn how much time it takes you to recover from the normal stress of things like walking to a neighborhood store, climbing a flight of stairs, etc.

Morning Pulse

More often than not, as you reach higher states of fitness, you will obtain correspondingly lower heart rate levels. This conditioning phenomenon can be easily observed by examining — and jotting down — your resting pulse throughout your yearly training program.

The best time to make this daily inquiry is after a long period of rest — specifically, just after waking up in the morning. What you will probably find, is that your morning pulse rate becomes lower after several months of regular training.

If your exercise program is not yielding lower morning pulse rate figures, it may indicate that you have reached a plateau in your health and fitness. A plateau is a natural juncture in every athlete's training cycle. In time — somewhere between 2 and 4 months — your heart rate will begin to decline again.

Some people, however, will observe a steady rise in their morning heart rate. Should this happen, it is usually a sign that their health and/or fitness are deteriorating. If the morning pulse remains significantly higher than normal, it calls for the reduction in intensity of an athlete's training program. Should this revision fail to have a positive effect, then it may be necessary to seek out a sports physician's help.

It is not uncommon to wake up one day and find your morning pulse to be markedly higher than usual. Assume, for example, that your normal morning pulse is 52 bpm. Then, out of the blue, your regular 8 AM reading jumps to 72 bpm. When this happens — and even world-class athletes experience such moments — it's typically an indicator that your body is being forced to work harder for some reason.

This unusual elevation in your normal morning pulse, then, provides an excellent opportunity to reflect on your current life situation. Maybe you are experiencing too much stress at home, on the job, or at school. Perhaps you are about to come down with a cold or the flu (two biochemical versions of a physical injury). Moreover, don't rule out the possibility that a soaring morning pulse could be a harbinger of a hidden stress — such as an impending injury from over-training.

Whenever your morning heart rate increases unexpectedly, it's wise to *stop, think, and respond quickly*. One appropriate response, as mentioned above, is to decrease the amount of time and the intensity of your scheduled workout. Another option — and only you can be the judge if this is necessary — is to eliminate that day's training session altogether. In all likelihood, either one of these conservative measures should bring your morning heart rate back to normal in a day or so.

Suppose, to bring your morning pulse back to normal, you elect not to exercise for some time — be it as little as one day or as long as two weeks. When you do resume your training program, it's important to take it easy at first. Don't try to overcompensate for 'lost' time or miles. Remember, your body and/or mind has just been through something. And a hasty effort to recover your form could precipitate the illness or injury you either had or just avoided.

By diligently monitoring and logging the morning pulse rate in a diary, you can become more sensitive to how you are feeling, both mentally and physically. Furthermore, this athletic journal will enable you to determine whether or not your fitness is improving.

Correlating Heart Rate, Speed, and Cadence

One of the most frequent questions asked by cyclists is what is the ideal pedaling rate, or cadence. Traditionalists usually suggest a figure that ranges anywhere from 90 to 120 revolutions per minute. This suggestion, which is crude at best, also fails to consider an individual rider's heart rate. A more accurate way to determine optimum cadence starts by asking a different question: How fast can you ride with the most efficiency at your lowest heart rate?

This very valuable information can be obtained in two ways. First, by using a HRM that measures speed, cadence, and heart rate. A second option is to employ a basic HRM along with a cyclocomputer. By adhering to the following method, you can plot a graph that shows how fast you should be spinning the cranks.

☐ Ride over the test course at your maximum speed, at your maximum aerobic heart rate. (For purpose of illustration, let's say you're able to travel 23 mph at 165 bpm, which puts you in the upper reaches of the target zone.)

☐ After the first test ride, give yourself adequate time to recover. How long this will take is determined by noting your active resting pulse — the number of heart bpm when walking, sitting, and standing — on the HRM. Try to relax during these moments. By concentrating on breathing rhythmically, you may be able to reduce your heart rate more rapidly. Indeed, this recovery technique can prove invaluable to racers.

☐ As soon as you have recovered, ride the test circuit at your maximum heart rate again. But this time shift-up one gear as you try to increase your speed.

☐ If you are able to go faster, repeat steps 2 and 3 until your speed levels off or begins dropping. If your rides and recovery times total 30–45 minutes, you will probably register lower speeds as well as lower heart rates. Should this occur, it will invalidate the accuracy of your test results. So, if your cadence research lasts one half to three quarters of an hour, stop and then resume it the next day.

☐ The test is over when you can no longer ride any faster. At this point, you have determined the most efficient cadence and gearing that will provide maximum speed while remaining in the target zone.

Once you have established these base figures, you might want to engage in further experimentation. Try adopting different handlebar positions (on the top, the brake levers and the drops), as well as saddle locations by sitting fore and aft. As you make each of these changes, pay close attention to your heart rate, speed, and cadence. This kind of fine-tuning will help optimize your cycling efficiency.

Aerobic Cycling Throughout the Yearly Training Program

Whether you are a novice or a veteran cyclist, the key to building and maintaining your aerobic base is increasing the amount of workout time. How much time you can spend exercising depends on your own particular circumstances: Each individual has a unique response to the physical stress of training, while personal commitments (work, family, school, etc.) also have to be taken into consideration. Given these fundamental provisos, some general rules will apply to most athletes:

☐ Regardless of how long you are able to exercise — whether 15 minutes or 5 hours — maintain that time frame for at least 2 weeks. This axiom should be adhered to before making any change in your training schedule. Staying with your current regimen for 14 days, before adding more time, gives your body an opportunity to adapt to new physical demands.

☐ In a training program that does not exceed 45 minutes, do not increase your training time — at any point — by more than 50 percent. If your training sessions are longer — say 1 hour — you can add 15 minute increments at 2-week intervals. This gradual incremental approach will enable your body to benefit from the increased workload.

☐ Clinical experience with novice, recreational, and world-class cyclists and triathletes demonstrates that each group feels most comfortable — physiologically and psychologically — when they reach one of three primary riding time levels within each category: 45 minutes, 60 minutes, and 90 minutes for the novice rider; 60 minutes, 90 minutes, and 2 hours for the seasoned fitness cyclist or racer; and 3 hours, 4 hours, and 5 hours for the elite athlete.

When you progress to any one of these essential levels, you should remain there for at least 4 weeks before adding more time to your training sessions.

You may be quite content to exercise no longer than 45 minutes — and that is quite acceptable. You will still be rewarded with health and fitness benefits — providing you exercise in the target zone 5 times per week.

☐ Should you experience any physical problem during this training program *stop* immediately. It's time to begin re-evaluating your exercise schedule. Frequently, aches and pains are a sign that you are doing too much too soon.

As both the beginner and veteran spend more time on the bicycle, they can, for example, experience knee pain during and after riding. If this happens, take a few days off. And when you do get back in the saddle, ride for a month only at the level where you were before you began to feel the discomfort. (This means that if you incurred knee pain upon moving your daily ride up from 1 hour to 1 hour and 15 minutes, your rides for the next month should not exceed 60 minutes.)

But should your pain either persist after spending several days not training, or return after you resume your scaled-down program, it's advisable to consult a sports physician. Being injured does not mean you should stop exercising. Rather, it means you have a physical problem that must be diagnosed and corrected promptly.

CHAPTER 6

Sample Training Programs

To get you started on the road to fitness and health, here are three introductory sample training programs geared to novice, intermediate, and advanced athletes, respectively. While these programs should be seen as practical examples that apply most specifically to cyclists, the same basic formats may be used by runners and swimmers, too. Table 6-1 summarizes the typical programs for the aerobic phase of training.

Each of these introductory training programs is designed to build up your aerobic base. Once you have accomplished this without experiencing any physical problems, you're ready to move on to the next stage. During this two-week period, you will be working on improving your aerobic speed.

Upon entering the aerobic speed phase, you are bridging the gap between casual exercise and outright training. Specifically, you will be spending more time riding:

☐ Once or twice a week, ride two times on the same day. During these AM and PM rides, stay in the lower range of your target zone.

☐ Once a week, ride 20 to 25 percent longer than any of your other workouts, making sure that your heart rate remains in the middle to upper ranges of the target zone.

With these two alterations in mind, your training schedule — depending on your level of ability — may look like the ones outlined in Table 6-2.

The day before your single longest ride should be spent off the bike, since it is essential to be well-rested to realize the maximum benefits from this longer workout. You should ride on the day after this effort — but be mindful to maintain a relatively slow cadence. Remaining active will help your body eliminate toxins.

Note to Table 6-1. Whatever your level of proficiency, starting your aerobic phase of training should almost feel too easy. These schedules, like the ones that follow, can be modified by adjusting the days and times to fit your specific needs. However, try to maintain the same order. For example, if Saturday is the busiest day of your week, slide the entire schedule one day to the right, giving you an 'off' day on Saturday, 30 minutes on Sunday, etc.

Table 6-1 Aerobic training phase

Novice:

Mon	Tues	Wed	Thurs	Fri	Sat	Sun
off*	30 min	20 min	30 min	off*	30 min	20 min

* For the beginner working a typical full time job, Monday and Friday are good 'off' days

Intermediate:

Mon	Tues	Wed	Thurs	Fri	Sat	Sun
60 min	90 min	60 min	90 min	60 min	off	120–150 min

Advanced:

Mon	Tues	Wed	Thurs	Fri	Sat	Sun
90 min	90 min	120 min	120 min	off	60 min	120–150 min

Aerobic Intervals

Although most people assume interval training always involves anaerobic efforts, that is not the case: It's quite possible to perform intervals and still remain within aerobic parameters. Aerobic intervals can be done in the latter part of your first or second Aerobic Base periods. And because these workouts allow for a smooth transition to anaerobic training, they are particularly useful in a competitive training program.

During the early phase of the Aerobic Base program, you may find it easy to achieve your MAF. Later on, as you ride faster upon approaching that level, you may experience a great degree of physical discomfort. More than likely, you'll perceive it as too hard to maintain that pace every day. As a result, you tend to work out at higher speeds — but at lower heart rates. When this happens, you're ready to begin aerobic intervals.

An aerobic interval can be as short as 3 to 5 minutes or as long 10 to 15 minutes. Whichever time span you select, be realistic: Make sure you can sustain a pace that will keep you at your maximum aerobic heart rate. Even though this type of interval can bring you well above your normal speed, the workout will still be aerobic.

Sample 90-Minute Aerobic Interval Work-Out

For the sample interval, let's suppose that you can only ride at your maximum aerobic level of 145 bpm for 3 to 5 minutes. This, then, is the length of your interval. (When performing intervals, stay within your prescribed time, rather than establishing a numerical objective, such as 5 sets.) After each interval — which can be performed on a course that is either hilly or flat — slow your pace down to a comfortable heart rate (125–135 bpm) for 6 to 10 minutes:

71

☐ 15 minute warm-up period.

☐ 3–5 minutes at your maximum aerobic heart rate (MAF), i.e. 145 bpm in this example.

☐ 6–10 minutes at a more comfortable pace, 10–20 bpm lower than your maximum heart rate, i.e. 125–135 bpm in this example.

☐ Continue alternating between the pace at which you reach your maximum aerobic heart rate (145 bpm) and the one at which the heart rate is 10–20 bpm lower (125–135 bpm) until the start of the cool-down period.

☐ Finish off with a 15-minute cool-down period.

Note to Table 6-2. As you progress in your aerobic phase, unless you're able to ride longer almost every day, it's a good idea to get a double workout once during the week. Even if one workout is indoors on a trainer, it can help stimulate the aerobic system and help you build a better base.

Table 6-2 Speed phase

Novice:

Mon	Tues	Wed	Thurs	Fri	Sat	Sun
off	45 min	45 min (am) 45 min (pm)	75 min	off	75 min	30 min

Intermediate:

Mon	Tues	Wed	Thurs	Fri	Sat	Sun
60 min	90 min	60 min (am) 60 min (pm)	90 min	120 min	off	3 hrs

Advanced:

Mon	Tues	Wed	Thurs	Fri	Sat	Sun
60–90 min	90 min	2 hrs	3 hrs	2 hrs	off	3–5 hrs

Anaerobic Training and Racing (April 1 to July 1)

During this period, you should do anywhere from one to three workouts per week that are designed to raise your heart rate above its Aerobic Maximum. Make no mistake, anaerobic training is extremely demanding. Yet all cyclists — even those who have no intention of competing — should include these workouts in their schedule. It's a matter of attaining bodily balance. Riders who fail to reach this equilibrium may incur poor health, lower levels of fitness, or a combination of these undesirable conditions.

Before scheduling your anaerobic sessions, it's worth considering the following guidelines:

☐ Typically, there should be at least 2, but no more than 3 anaerobic workouts per week.

☐ The day before an anaerobic effort should either be an *off* day on your training schedule or it should be used for easy, aerobic riding.

☐ Don't forget to warm-up and cool-down thoroughly on the days you perform your anaerobic routines.

☐ Anaerobic workouts should never be done on consecutive days.

☐ The day following this intense effort should find you taking a short ride at an easy aerobic pace.

☐ A race is considered an anaerobic workout.

☐ The anaerobic period is minimally 5 weeks in duration, assuming you don't experience any physical problems. Maximally, it should not go beyond 12–15 weeks.

☐ You are clearly anaerobic when your heart rate is above its Aerobic Maximum level. And, generally, if you are either mildly anaerobic or have reached your highest anaerobic

Note to Table 6-3. Once you progress to the anaerobic phase, drop in those harder workouts on the most stress-free days. For most people, twice weekly is enough. If you compete, one of those anaerobic workouts can be an actual race. For the most advanced, three anaerobic days is the maximum. Never have two anaerobic days back to back.

Table 6-3 Anaerobic training phase

Novice:

Mon	Tues	Wed	Thurs	Fri	Sat	Sun
off or easy spin	Anaerobic: 15 min warm-up 30-45 min anaer., 15 min cool-down	45 min	30 min	off	Anaerobic: 15 min warm-up 45-60 anaer. 15 min cool-down	45 min

Intermediate:

Mon	Tues	Wed	Thurs	Fri	Sat	Sun
60 min	Anaerobic: 15 min warm-up 60 min anaerobic 15 min cool-down	60 min	120 min	90 min	60n min	Anaerobic: 30 min warm-up 2 hrs anaer. 30 min cool-down or race

Advanced:

Mon	Tues	Wed	Thurs	Fri	Sat	Sun
60-90 min	Anaerobic: 30 min warm-up 2 hrs anaerobic 15 min on/off 30 min cool-down	60-90 min	Anaerobic same as Tues	60-90 min	60-90: min	3-5 hrs or race

state, many of the benefits are similar. Therefore, when you are doing anaerobic workouts, your pulse should not exceed your average competitive heart rate by more than 5 to 8 percent. (Competitive heart rate is highly individual, since it's an undefined number of bpm above a racer's target zone.) If you drive your pulse beyond this quotient, you are not only wasting energy, but running the risk of overtraining as well.

Sample anaerobic programs for each level of proficiency are listed in Table 6-3.

Intervals

Anaerobic Intervals can be executed either in the hills or on the flats, so long as you abide by the guideline listed under the last point above: Don't exceed your competitive pulse rate by more than 5 to 8 percent. The only cyclists exempted from this caveat are those racers who are attempting to improve their sprinting techniques. Usually, sprinting in a race demands an all-out effort for no more than 500 meters. And, during this short burst, it's highly impractical not to permit your heart rate to rise above the 5 to 8 percent boundary. But even burly-thighed sprinters must be careful not to push themselves beyond a certain limit.

Let's say that 8 percent above your competitive heart rate lies between 175 and 180 bpm. After 4 sets of sprint intervals, your pulse has been consistently in this range. It's a good bet that you have already obtained the maximum fitness benefits from your workout—and to ride another set could harm your body.

As you continue on with anaerobic training, the HRM will tell you whether or not you're making fitness advances. Assume, for instance, that your maximum heart rate rises to 180 bpm at the beginning of your interval practice. There are two ways of gauging your progress after a month or two of performing these workouts.

First, you can consistently demonstrate the ability to complete your interval sets at the same times — over the same distance — at lower heart rates. A second, and even better, indication of your improving fitness is this: You can perform your interval sets in faster times, over the same distance, at the same heart rate — in this case 180 bpm.

Sometimes, your heart rate may increase, or your times may get slower when doing interval workouts. When this happens, you should ask yourself the following questions:

☐ Have you made a mistake in your calculations and come up with too high a figure for your maximum heart rate?

☐ Are you performing too many intervals during a session?

☐ Have you gone beyond the recommended number of days for your interval program?

☐ Are you doing too much anaerobic training in general?

☐ Are you failing to consume enough fluids during these demanding efforts?

In all likelihood, if you responded *Yes* to any or all of these questions, you will have discovered the source(s) of your declining speed and/or rising heart rate. Some adjustment(s), therefore, will be necessary.

Weight Training

Weight training, according to most bicycle training manuals, should be performed during the off season. This is incorrect. Pumping iron, because it demands that your muscles produce both power and strength, is clearly an anaerobic exercise. This is true whether you are doing numerous light weight repetitions or fewer repetitions with the really heavy metal.

The HRM has two primary functions during weight lifting sessions. It will remind you to warm-up and cool-down thoroughly as well as ensure that your recovery time between sets is sufficient.

Throughout the weight workout itself, heart rate is not a valid means of distinguishing aerobic from anaerobic. That's because, in this instance, your pulse will reach a plateau very quickly. Yet, before this happens, the repetitions are over — or, more precisely, your muscles fatigue and you stop lifting. As a result, you don't obtain an accurate reading from the HRM due to the short time you are actually exercising.

The one exception to this assertion applies to the novice athlete who has just started a training program. In this case, if you should lift weights, your heart rate will rise rapidly and may exceed its aerobic maximum before finishing the workout. Novices are better off concentrating on building an aerobic base, and that objective will not be achieved by lifting weights.

Aerobic Base Period (A Break from Anaerobic Training and Racing), July 1 to August 15

The value of the second Aerobic Base Period for competitive cyclists is twofold. First, it helps them recoup some of their energies expended on races during the spring and early summer. Second, this break can enable racers to peak for the big events that frequently close out their racing calendar. For the fitness enthusiast, this period is a welcome respite from the strain of performing intense, anaerobic interval workouts.

If you ride to stay in shape, you will probably experience no difficulty in making this transition. Racers, however, may find that this second Aerobic Base Period does pose some logistical problems. Often, due to the complexity and fullness of their competitive program, it will be hard to set aside the time to adequately recharge their aerobic system. To avoid missing out on this important training phase, racers should take time at the beginning of the season to factor this period into the yearly calendar.

Resumption of Anaerobic Training and Racing, August 1 to November 15

Throughout this 3½-month period, both the competitive and fitness cyclist should repeat the sequence of exercises outlined in the first anaerobic segment. This is an opportune moment to make any needed adjustments in your training plan.

This is where your training diary will come in very handy. If you have been faithfully recording and entering your morning pulse rate, along with your workout and/or competition data, you can easily determine whether you are progressing, regressing, or plateauing. But before modifying your workout schedule, make the following investigation:

☐ Is your morning heart rate consistently higher, lower, or stable?

☐ Throughout your day, do you feel that you have more or less energy?

☐ Have you been free of injury and illness? Or have you been caught in a web of colds and the flu, and/or experiencing some serious aches and pains?

☐ Are the times on your test course during MAF-test rides higher, lower, or remaining constant?

☐ How are you performing during Aerobic Interval workouts — faster, slower, or unchanged?

☐ When doing Anaerobic Intervals, is your heart rate higher, lower, or stable? Is your speed holding steady, or are you riding faster or slower?

☐ If you have been racing, it's important to consider your level of experience. Usually, novice racers can't expect to make the same gains as their savvy counterparts. Bearing this in mind, do you see any changes in your performance? Are you getting more or fewer top-10 finishes? Are you coming in with the bunch, or ending up in 'no man's land'? Are you able to cover the crucial breaks, or are you getting dropped? Do you have the strength to initiate attacks? When the race enters the hills, can you stay up front with leaders, or do you become a caboose?

Upon carefully appraising your responses, you will know whether or not to use this second anaerobic period to maintain or modify your training regimen.

The ideal training program should promote your health as well as your conditioning. This means you should not engage in any activities that could compromise your well-being in exchange for potential fitness benefits. In truth, if you follow a course that keeps this principle in mind, you can establish complete body harmony.

CHAPTER 7

Competition

A heart rate monitor is extremely beneficial for athletes who engage in competition. By periodically noting their heart rates during a race, they can conserve precious energy as well as maximize performance.

Whatever kind of race you compete in, it's only natural that your heart rate will be constantly yo-yoing upward and downward. An all-out sprint, for example, obviously will send your pulse rate rocketing skyward; while sitting in the pack for an extended period of time could find your pulse rate numbers plummeting below the target zone. This kind of ebbing and flowing of your heart rate is very costly from an energy conservation standpoint. Most significantly, it saps your stamina and, ultimately, causes fatigue to come on quicker.

Figure 5.4, in Chapter 5, shows the heart rate of a competitor throughout a race: Ideally, you want to maintain a pace that allows you to maintain a steady heart rate throughout the event. Sometimes, this may seem impossible — as when climbing a very steep hill, for example. Yet, if you moderate your efforts on a demanding gradient, you can expect to gain some advantages over your opponents later in the race. Your heart rate will remain within the target zone's parameters and, consequently, you will have more strength left when approaching the finish line.

Usually, racers who are not strong climbers are reluctant to adopt a less than all-out strategy. They feel that holding back on an ascent will cause them to lose contact with either the peloton or the lead group. If you don't have the kind of legs that allow you to dance up mountains, you will do well to adopt traditional bike racing tactics.

Before the race, scout the course and learn where the major climbs are located. Then, during the event, as you approach each ascent, move to the front of the group you are riding with. As you begin climbing, make sure you sustain a rhythm that keeps you within the target zone. Frequently, this very basic maneuver may serve to either cut your losses or keep you up with the race leaders. What is almost certain, however, is that you will have conserved a lot of energy — which can be utilized after you crest the summit.

Commonly, those racers who go beyond their target zone's upper limit during a gut-busting ascent, have to coast down, freewheeling to recover on the descent. But by riding within the competitive target zone, you will have another option: You can shift into a higher gear and begin charging down the hill.

The Individual and Team Time Trial

A heart rate monitor is a boon to riders who plan to enter either an individual or a team time trial. During training rides, you can use it in conjunction with a stopwatch to improve your form and evaluate your equipment. Wearing a HRM on practice runs will help determine the ideal saddle position to keep you in the target zone. Furthermore, you can use the device to evaluate which handlebars, crank lengths, wheels, helmet, clothing, and even which bike will save you precious seconds during a race — which will pay of on the day of the race.

When it comes to the target zone during a competive time trial, you do not have to be all that concerned about the upper limit of your pulse rate. That is because you should primarily be concerned with squeezing out every drop of energy from the human engine. In time trials, you should be neither surprised nor worried if you are able to push your heart rate above its normal maximum.

Yet, in order to get the most out of your body during this 'race of truth,' pay close attention to the HRM when warming up. Take at least 15 minutes to raise your heart rate to its highest aerobic level. Then maintain a pace that pegs the pulse at this figure for another 10 to 15 minutes. Follow this up with several short sprints and recoveries which allows your pulse rate to drop just below the target zone. The virtue of this warm-up routine will be evident soon after the event begins: In just a few minutes, you should be able to comfortably pedal at your racing cadence.

The Stage Race

During a stage race, cyclists are going through a very unique situation. For several days — or weeks — they find themselves continuously preparing for competition, expending energy, and recovering. Using a HRM as a bio-feedback unit, can help you achieve your best results throughout these physically and mentally demanding contests.

Regardless of a stage race's duration, an intelligent rider must formulate a strategy. This strategy, however, goes beyond fundamental cycling tactics. In order to be successful — as well as survive the ordeal — you have to pay careful attention to your body. Observing your heart rate from morning to night can help you decide whether this is a day to hold back or to attack.

When competing in a multi-day event, it's crucial to check your morning pulse rate on a daily basis. Just as in training, this figure is an accurate barometer of your physical condition. Be aware of the fact that, as you spend day after day at or above your maximum aerobic pace (MAP), there will be a corresponding rise in your morning heart rate. Still, if you happen to notice a sharp rise in your heart rate upon waking up, try to play it conservatively during the day's event. On the other hand, if you are in really good form, your morning pulse may be the same as usual. When you record such readings, you can approach the day's stage with the well-founded confidence that your body possesses a sufficient amount of energy in reserve.

At the race's onset, keep your eye on your HRM. Invariably, after many miles of pedaling, you will see a rise in your pulse rate. If you notice that you're riding slower and inefficiently while in the target zone, it's a sign that your body is not feeling strong. Therefore this is not the time for aggressive cycling. Instead, sit-in for as long as possible, conserving your energy for the race's key breakaway. But let's say you can comfortably maintain your pace with pulse rate numbers that lie in the lower portion of the target zone. This is a good indication that your body has ample energy and, should the opportunity present itself, you could go on the offensive.

After the day's competition is completed, don't forget to monitor your daytime resting pulse rate. This will provide you with valuable information about your recovery process. From observing your heart rate after hard training rides and single-day races, you should be thoroughly aware of how your body responds to the stress placed upon it. If you are obtaining your usual numbers upon finishing a stage, there's no need to alter the strategy you have planned for the next day. However, should you see that the resting pulse is higher than normal, it's advisable to moderate your effort during the next day of racing.

By monitoring your heart rate before, during, and after every stage, you can enhance your performance and minimize the chance of injury and/or illness.

Irrespective of the competitive event, many racers make an all too common mistake: They ride too fast relative to their ability. Although this is understandable, given the psychological investment most riders have made in winning, you can reach more of your potential by not going all out at the sound of the starter's pistol. Be aware of your heart rate for the first few miles, making sure you remain in the lower portion of the target zone. This conservative approach will enable you to ride within yourself. Unfortunately, while many racers understand this principle, they have quite a lot of difficulty putting it into practice.

Competition Recommendations

The purpose of these recommendations is to allow your body and mind to function optimally. And on the day of a big race, who doesn't want that to happen? The means to achieving this highly desirable end is to eliminate much of the structural, chemical, and mental stresses a racer experiences before, during, and after competition.

The Week Before the Race

All right, you've been very disciplined. For the past several months you have scrupulously adhered to your training regimen. Consequently, with a contest only 7 days away, you know that you have the mental and physical capabilities that could result in a top-10 placing — or a possible victory. But even if you are in peak condition, you can still turn in a terrible performance by failing to follow any one of several pre-race guidelines.

Generally, the body doesn't like to go through severe changes. So don't change any of the positive habits you have formed throughout the yearly training plan during the week leading up to your event. Yet, in order to fine-tune your conditioning, specific modifications will be necessary:

☐ In the week preceding the competition, slightly decrease your regular cycling mileage. Make sure, too, that all your rides are relatively easy ones. The exception to this, however, is when your fitness schedule calls for riding anaerobically. In this instance, limit yourself to one hard effort four days before the race.

☐ Being in great physical shape alone doesn't guarantee a good competitive performance. The mind also comes into play. Remember, you do have control over your thoughts. Try to ignore subconscious negative tape-loops. ("I'm afraid he/she is much better than I am;" "I really can't do this;" etc.) As each day brings the race closer, become more mentally focused on the impending effort. Be optimistic but realistic. Maintaining a balanced psychological state, indeed, can effect your race results.

The Day Before the Race: To Ride or Not to Ride?

Many cyclists perform better when they don't ride on the day before a race. Depending on how your body feels, as well as your level of confidence, two days off might also be appropriate. Don't be afraid to experiment with these suggestions — however, putting in the miles at the 'twelfth hour' is really of no benefit. Still, if you're tense before the event, you might take your bike out for an easy spin. Be aware of the fact that even professional riders experience some anxiety prior to an important race. It's all right to be a little edgy before your event — and knowing how to manage this emotion can be an invaluable asset.

CHAPTER 8

Race Care: Before, During and After the Event

This chapter is devoted to providing athletes with information on some of the important aspects that are only too often overlooked before, during and after competition. You can improve your race results and promote your recuperation process significantly by adhering to these simple instructions.

What to Eat — And Not to Eat — the Day Before the Race

☐ Don't eat shellfish: that includes shrimp, lobster, clams, mussels, scallops, or any other similar creatures of the sea. Commonly, people have adverse reactions to shellfish in stressful situations and your pre-race day definitely qualifies as one of those times. Incidentally, shellfish are highly toxic and you will be producing more than enough toxins on your own, in the form of lactic acid.

☐ Don't eat raw and other foods that are difficult to digest. That means avoiding nuts, seeds, black pepper, corn (including popcorn), as well as uncooked fruits and vegetables. (Avocado is an exception on this proscribed list, since it contains lipase, an enzyme that promotes fat metabolism, thus inproving your endurance.) Since you are probably in a mild, if not a major, state of stress, your intestinal tract has become less efficient. Eating salads and the like at such moments could bring on stomach problems.

☐ If you don't normally consume alcoholic beverages, don't get caught up in the usual pre-race festivities. But, if you usually enjoy small amounts of beer or wine with your food, then continue on with this mealtime ritual. A glass or two of your preferred drink is an aid to digestion and helps your fatty acid metabolism which improves endurance.

Don't drink bottle after bottle of beer, thinking that it is a good way of hydrating yourself. Overdoing the hops will have the opposite effect. Some people cannot tolerate beer's carbonation. Should you be one of these folks but want to drink anyway, switch over to wine.

☐ Whole-grains should be part of your daily diet in general, so continue eating them right up to the competition. A high-quality carbohydrate meal — such as whole-grain pasta or brown rice topped with cooked vegetables — makes an excellent pre-race dinner. Polishing off a desert is also acceptable. Just don't eat large amounts of refined carbohydrates (sugar), thinking that to do so will help you perform better. It won't.

☐ Try not to eat your pre-race dinner after 8 PM. Your intestinal tract is very inefficient late in the evening.

☐ About an hour and a half after you have eaten dinner, begin drinking small amounts of water (about 4 ounces) every 30 minutes to hydrate yourself. Continue this procedure right up until bedtime. If you don't have access to a tap at all times, fill up one or two water bottles and take them with you.

Travel Recommendations

If you are lucky, you won't have to travel more than an hour or so to get to the city or town where the race is held. But sooner or later you may be faced with a lengthy journey by car, plane, or train, as well as staying in a hotel or motel and eating in restaurants. All of these circumstances present logistic problems. And how you deal with them can truly effect your competitive performance.

☐ When traveling to your destination by plane, be aware of the fact that the cabin is pressurized and low in humidity. In this atmosphere, your oxygen uptake will be lower; and since the body tends to lose moisture, you may become mildly dehydrated. On flights lasting under two hours, these are not very significant problems. During longer trips, however, it is important not to ignore such matters. Fortunately, the remedy is as simple as continually drinking small amounts of water. You can avoid walking about the craft by keeping a water bottle at your seat.

☐ During very long flights, it's a good idea to get out of your seat periodically and take a stroll up and down the isle. Sitting too long in a cramped space could cause your body to become stiff.

☐ Airplane cuisine is probably just a step up from hospital food. So it's best to avoid it if this is at all possible.

☐ Regardless of how many flights you have logged, when traveling by plane your sympathetic nervous system functions at a higher rate than normal (this is an adrenal response to the stress of flying). Consequently, the intestinal tract loses some of its digestive efficiency. If you become hungry and want to eat in mid-flight, here are some foods to skip: raw fruits and vegetables, nuts, seeds, popcorn, and black pepper. All of these products are difficult to digest when you are airborne.

☐ If you dislike airplane food, or you don't eat meat, all is not lost. Call the airline at least 24 hours before your scheduled departure and order a meal that comes the closest to your usual dietary regimen. Should you happen to be a vegetarian, more than likely the alternative menu will include raw vegetables which, remember, are hard on the digestive system. The best way out of this situation is to carry your own food aboard the airplane.

☐ Coffee drinkers should keep their cups to a minimum as this beverage inhibits proper intestinal functioning.

☐ Just because the airline may serve complimentary wine, beer, or cocktails, doesn't mean that you're dutybound to accept any. In a low pressurized cabin alcohol becomes highly potent.

Traveling by Car

For the bicycle racer, the automobile offers the widest range of travel options. You can bring an abundance of your favorite snacks and have picnic meals — plus you can stop whenever you want and walk around in the fresh air. However, traveling by car can be fatiguing. If your race site is at a considerable distance, try to arrive the day before the event. This will allow your body time to recover from the long hours — or days — spent on the road.

Accommodations

☐ After you have dumped all your gear on the hotel or motel room floor and tested the bed, check out the available water source. If it isn't to your taste, make non-carbonated, bottled spring water the the first item on your shopping list. Add to that enough of your preferred food snacks. While you're jotting down items, consider whether you are planning to eat a pre-race breakfast or lunch. Even if there is a restaurant adjacent to your accommodations, it's not very likely that breakfast will be served early enough to permit adequate digestion. (e.g. 6 AM on a Sunday). And even if you're fortunate enough to find an establishment that is open, obtaining a nourishing meal might be difficult. You may be able to avoid these hassles and associated tensions if your room is equipped with some basic cooking facilities.

☐ Seasoned travelers know the value of opening their room's window(s) in order to have fresh air circulating. Usually, in modern hotels this is impossible, since the windows are hermetically sealed. Faced with this situation, switch the fan on to its lowest setting. Should the room become hot and/or humid, set the air conditioner at a comfortable minimum.

☐ Getting a good night's sleep can make a tremendous difference in how you feel and perform on race day. Although there may be some hot parties happening, pass them up and go to bed early. Even if you can't sleep, you won't be needlessly squandering energy.

Race Day

☐ As soon as you wake up and are out of bed, drink a large glass of water. This helps eliminate bodily wastes and begins your hydration process.

☐ Allow time to perform your normal morning rituals: taking a shower, going to the toilet, reading the paper, etc.

☐ If you're entered in an early morning event that is not too long (an 8 AM race, 25 miles in length is a good example), you may not need to eat breakfast. A race that is held later in the day, or one that is considerably longer, definitely requires you to have a morning meal. Follow the guidelines listed below for the morning meal:

1. Have your meal at least 1½ to 2½ hours before the start of the race.

2. Steer clear of foods and beverages containing concentrated carbohydrates (sugars): jellies, doughnuts, candy, fruit, fruit juices, and soda, as well as energy replacement drinks that contain more than 3 percent sugar. Including any of these items on your race day menu will inhibit fats and, hence, your endurance. When much needed fats are decreased, your body is forced to rely on glucose. It's crucial to keep glucose in reserve so it's available during the key parts of the race.

3. An appropriate race day meal can be as small as a slice or two of whole wheat toast or as large as two eggs — without the whites — along with those bread products. Another nourishing option is oatmeal with a small amount of butter. Avoid milk: if you are feeling tense, it can upset your stomach.

☐ Coffee: Many cyclists like to drink a cup or two of coffee before a race. Indeed, this practice will raise the level of fatty acid in the blood, which is highly desirable. Yet the same result can be attained by a proper warm-up. It's advisable, then, to allow your body to reach this state naturally, without relying on caffeine (a drug, albeit a legal one in a specified dosage). If, however, you choose to include coffee in your diet, here is some information to take into consideration:

a. Coffee has a dehydrating effect, so if you drink it, you will need to take in more water before, during, and after the race.

b. Coffee will begin producing negative effects on your body after about two hours upon its consumption. Therefore, if you are going to drink this beverage, do so at least 30 minutes before the race. Should you be racing for more than 1½ hours, it's advisable not to consume any coffee.

c. If you must imbibe this beverage, don't use milk or sugar.

d. Some racers feel that coffee perks them up psychologically. However, if you require a drug to get into this mental space, it may be a sign of a lack of confidence.

☐ Make sure you get to the race site early enough to allow for a thorough warm-up. The pre-race warm-up is the key to achieving your potential during competition.

☐ After putting on your HRM, stay in the small chainring and spin slowly for 25 to 35 minutes. Gradually increase the pace, keeping your heart rate just below the target zone.

☐ Shift into the large chainring and, for no more than 10 minutes, do some short, race-pace sprints. This should bring your heart rate into the target zone.

Once the Race Begins

☐ Whether the temperature is 40 or 100 degrees F (4 and 37°C respectively), most racers will begin to dehydrate after 10 to 12 minutes of hard riding. A rule of thumb, then, is that whether or not you feel thirsty, consume water from your bottle every 15 minutes. At this ratio, a standard water bottle should last nearly one hour.

☐ By glancing at the HRM, you may note that your pulse rate begins to rise as the need for water increases.

☐ At the risk of sounding obvious, you must be able to drink water while speeding along on your bicycle. If you have difficulty doing this, practice drinking water at a high cadence on your test course.

☐ Don't drink ice water. It's too cold for your stomach to handle. Despite the fact that cold water (41 °F, or 5 °C) empties from the stomach quite quickly, it also creates the possibility of cramping.

☐ It's very easy for unhealthy microbes to grow in old water bottles. And when there is a significant accumulation, they can make you sick while you're racing. Purchase a set of bottles that are strictly reserved for competition — and keep them spotlessly clean inside.

☐ In races that last longer than two hours, your body may deplete more elements than just water. Some cyclists may exhaust certain electrolytes in the latter stages of their event. (Usually sodium is depleted first, but potassium and calcium are also quickly consumed.) Therefore, during a particularly long and grueling competition, it may be necessary to take some of these nutrients.

Fluid Loss and Competition

Fluid loss and its replacement during competition — or while training — is an important consideration for most cyclists. The fluid most commonly depleted by all riders is water. Races that last up to two hours in duration usually only require replacing this liquid. This is especially the case for the rider who is both healthy and fit.

The Pre-Race Routine

Any fluid replacement beverage with a sugar content in excess of 3 percent will inhibit fat metabolism if consumed before the race. For the cyclist, this produces a pair of unwanted results. First, there is a loss of endurance; second, the body loses its ability to use fats for energy and, therefore, it has to rely on sugar. Since sugar, compared to fats, can provide the body with energy for only a relatively short time, this can cause the racer to literally run out of fuel before completing an event.

The reason an energy drink can cause a cyclist to lose stamina relates to the product's sugar content. A high concentration of sugar causes insulin to be released by the pancreas. This, in turn, prevents the body from using fats for fuel. In time, the blood sugar drops and there is a corresponding increase in the heart rate. As a consequence of this metabolic process, the body possesses neither enough sugar nor fats for energy. Because the aerobic system is so dependent on fats, a sugary energy replacement drink is a highly inefficient fuel.

If you consume a sugared drink prior to a race, you shouldn't be surprised if you bonk, or run out of strength. That's because when the utilization of fat is inhibited, the body is unable to spare, or save sugar. These sugar stores, which have a limited capacity, will be depleted long before you pass under the finish line banner.

Should you choose to dirnk an energy replacement drink anyway, make sure to check out its sugar content. If the percentage is above 3 percent, dilute it with water to lower this quotient — ideally it should have a 2.5 percent glucose content. Failure to reduce glucose to acceptable levels increases your chances of bonking.

Since you probably do not have access to a lab to measure how much glucose a beverage contains, you will have to rely on the taste test. A 2.5 percent glucose solution tastes like one teaspoon of table sugar in a 7 ounce glass of water. If you choose to drink soda or orange juice, you will have to employ a different mixing formula: An 8 ounce container of these fluids requires 25 ounces of water to dilute it to to an approximate 2.5 percent glucose concentration.

The Post-Race Routine

☐ As soon as you have completed your event, start drinking water — without ice. If the day has been hot and/or humid, sprinkle cool water over your body. Drinking a liquid containing about 80–100 grams of carbohydrate, such as maltodextrin, will greatly help recovery. Then towel off and put on some clean, dry clothes.

☐ After you have cooled down, go for an easy spin on the bike — or take a walk in sneakers or flip-flops — for 15 to 25 minutes.

☐ If you feel hungry after the race, the ideal food to eat is vegetable soup. It will immediately replace the most important minerals your body has lost without putting any stress on the intestinal system. If you are not competing too far from home, you could make your own vegetable soup and bring it to the event.

☐ Do not, under any circumstances, drink any alcohol for at least two hours upon completing a race. And eat something first before you do drink alcohol after that time. You are already in a dehydrated state, and beverages containing alcohol can leave you intoxicated or sick.

☐ Don't consume any products containing refined carbohydrates — sugary pastries, doughnuts or cookies — until after re-hydrating yourself with water and putting some nourishing food into your stomach. (The only exception to this stricture is in the case of a medical emergency. Should this happen, let trained medical personnel decide what is good for you and what is not.)

☐ Just completing your event — regardless of where you finish — is really a cause for celebration. This doesn't imply that you should begin partying or get drunk. Rather, it means chilling out a little in order to unwind from the tension of racing. By being kind and gentle to your body, it will perform better in competitive and non-competitive situations alike.

CHAPTER 9

Running and Swimming

As mentioned in earlier chapters, cyclists of all levels can derive health as well as fitness benefits from running and swimming. And since both of these exercise activities are fundamentally aerobic, swimmers and runners will definitely profit by training with a HRM.

Athletes who plan on focusing all of their energies on either running or swimming should adopt the same Yearly Training Plan as cyclists. Like two-wheel athletes, they must attain a balance between health and fitness by incorporating aerobic base periods with anaerobic workouts and/or competition.

MAF-Test for Runners

As you become a more proficient runner, the time and intensity of your workout will become greater. Running with a HRM, in the target zone, ensures that as the training demands increase, the stress on your body will remain constant.

Here's how this works: Let's say, for the purpose of illustration, that you are able to run 3 miles in 27 minutes, keeping your heart rate in a target zone of 130 bpm. Two months later, it's quite possible that you will be able to run the same distance — at the same heart rate — in about 25 minutes and 30 seconds.

Runners, like cyclists, can measure their aerobic progression through the self-administration of the MAF-test. When it comes to conducting the MAF-test, a runner has it somewhat easier than a bike rider. That's because an important variable

— the bicycle — has been eliminated. Moreover, this makes the test for running a bit more accurate, since the freewheeling, or coasting, factor is not applicable to the activity. However, other previously mentioned issues, such as climate, mental and physical states, etc., must still be taken into consideration.

The best location to perform the MAF-test is a quarter mile (or 400 meter) track. This facility will be easier to find than a velodrome, since your local high school or college probably has one. If locating a track does prove impossible, measure out a 'user-friendly' loop or stretch of road that is one mile long.

Upon arriving at your test course, begin by warming up for 10 to 15 minutes. At the end of this time, your heart rate should reach the lower threshold of the target zone. You are now ready to begin running at your maximum aerobic level.

With your HRM in the stopwatch mode, see how much time it takes to cover a mile at your maximum aerobic level. If you are able to maintain this pace for 5 miles — and don't go beyond this distance — clock each mile separately, and mentally record the figures. Should you be unable to sustain your aerobic maximum for 5 miles, then only run 2 miles, making sure to note your split times. Perform the MAF-test once every 3 weeks. This will provide concrete information as to whether you are progressing, plateauing, or regressing.

Table 9.1 Sample MAF-Test pattern

Mile	Time
I	9:00
2	9:12
3	9:18
4	9:25
5	9:38

As you perform the MAF-test, you will probably see the time for each subsequent mile gradually increase. This is normal, due to accumulated fatigue. If you run the first mile in 9 minutes, for example, the second mile may take 9 minutes and 12 seconds to cover. A typical MAF-test pattern looks like the one illustrated in Table 9-1.

Generally, in a 5-mile MAF-test, the difference in time between mile 1 and mile 5 should not be more than 45 to 60 seconds. If the differences in your test results exceed this time span, it usually means that running this distance is creating more stress than your body can tolerate. The best response to this situation is to restrict your MAF test to 2 miles.

Some runners who take the 5-mile test may find that their times for the first two miles are exactly the same, or they are able to run the second mile at a higher speed than the first one. The implication of either of these results is the need for a longer warm-up period. (The same inference can be made when such times are recorded during the 2-mile MAF-test.)

As you continue with your running program, you should begin to see gradual improvements in your maximum aerobic efficiency. By employing a HRM, you can objectively determine whether or not you are progressing. The training diary entries of a runner who is making gains commonly looks

Table 9-2 Sample training diary entries

Month	Heart Rate bpm	MAF (Mile Pace)
1	135	9:48
2	135	9:21
3	135	9:01
4	135	8:55
5	135	8:40

something like those summarized in Table 9-2. The two significant features in this log are the progressively faster times for the run and a stable heart rate.

As the months pass and your maximum aerobic efficiency improves, you will reach a point where your test times level off. There's no need for any concern. You simply have reached a natural plateau. What this means is that you have obtained the maximum aerobic benefits of the base period, and it's appropriate to begin your anaerobic workouts.

It's not uncommon to reach your aerobic peak several weeks before you are scheduled to begin anaerobic training. When this happens, it's wise to disregard the calendar — or else your body could become anaerobically deficient.

Anaerobic Workouts

Whether you are training for short or long distance races, eventually you should get on the track and perform interval workouts. During these gasp-inducing efforts, the HRM's primary function is to ensure that your recovery is adequate. A quick glance at the monitor after each interval dash will inform you when you're ready to go again.

Using a HRM in this manner flies in the face of the traditional approach of doing intervals. Customarily, runners conform to the following routine: They pound the track at their race pace for a quarter of mile and then jog for 220 yards. This format — which can continue for 30 to 45 minutes — revolves around the assumption that each 220 yard jog brings runners back to their recovery point. While this may work for some athletes, others find this recovery procedure unsatisfactory.

By employing a HRM, you can practice two other interval methods that will make your recovery period — as well as the rest of this workout — more effective:

☐ After warming up, perform a quarter mile interval at your anaerobic speed. Anaerobic speed is slightly faster than your racing pace and should not exceed your maximum aerobic heart rate by more than 15 percent (if you are training correctly, these two factors should coincide). Upon completing the interval, slow down and begin jogging. As you jog, keep an eye on the HRM. You will be ready to run your next anaerobic interval when your pulse drops just below your aerobic range.

Case History: Peter's Plateau

Peter was an extremely fit runner, who after following a training program he had read in a running magazine, seemed to reach a plateau in performance. His 5-kilometer times were stuck at around 16 minutes and he began to require 10 hours of sleep each night — but was still tired all day. Furthermore, he was coming down with a cold every 3 months, almost like clockwork.

All of these circumstances led Peter to consult a sports medicine doctor. He explained that his pace was close to 6 minutes per mile on easy training days, and nearly 1 minute faster during harder workouts. When the physician asked Peter to perform the MAF-test for 3 miles, he recorded times of 7:41, 7:49, and 7:58.

Given these results, Peter was advised to use a HRM while working out in an effort to slow down his pace. Shortly after employing this device, his aerobic training time progressed to 6:05, which enabled him to run a 5 kilometer race in 15:30 — a personal best. Better yet, he no longer needed as much sleep, while his energy and health reached a new peak.

If your pulse doesn't fall, or remains in the target zone for more than a minute, it means you did the anaerobic interval much too rapidly: Slow down!

As you proceed with the anaerobic workout, you will probably find that the time it takes to jog and recover will become progressively longer. This is a normal response to the intensity of anaerobic activity. When you find that your recovery requires the same time and/or distance as the interval itself, you have achieved the maximum benefits from the workout. At this point, begin cooling down.

☐ The second anaerobic interval method is based solely on time and heart rate. Because of this, you can do these workouts either on the road or on the track. After warming up, perform an interval for a specific period of time — say 1 minute. Then jog for as long as it takes to bring your heart rate just below its maximum aerobic range. When this occurs, repeat the interval. Continue this procedure for no more than 45 minutes, or until the interval and recovery times are almost the same. Some runners will adapt better to this format, since they are neither distracted by the necessity of counting laps nor bound by the imposition of a specified distance.

As you proceed through the anaerobic period, you will find that your maximum aerobic efficiency remains at a peak level. And, upon resuming aerobic base training again, you will be able to achieve even faster MAF-test times.

Maximum Aerobic Efficiency and its Relationship to Competition

There is a clear relationship between maximum aerobic efficiency and your ability to perform at a specific competitive pace for specified distances. A case study of a runner's maximum aerobic pace (MAP) — the first column in the chart — and race pace — the second column — is indicated in Table 9-3.

The significance of this example is that it demonstrates that the runner has achieved an excellent balance between health and fitness during his competitive period. If you are not obtaining similar results, it may be an indication that your body is either structurally or chemically imbalanced. Again, remedial action is called for. Start by re-evaluating your training program and life style. If this fails to correct the problem, it's advisable to seek out medical assistance.

But suppose you are able to complete your MAF-test run in 8 minutes — and can race a 5 km course in close to 18 minutes (a time that is better than a 5:30 pace per mile). While you might be pleased with this competitive outing, it really

Table 9-3 Race Pace Predicted

MAP per mile	5 km Race per mile	Time
10:00	7:30	23:18
9:00	7:00	21:45
8:30	6:45	20:58
8:00	6:30	20:12
7:30	6:00	18:38
7:00	5:30	17:05
6:30	5:15	16:19
6:00	5:00	15:32
5:45	4:45	14:45
5:30	4:30	13:59
5:00	4:20	13:28
5:00	4:15	13:12

isn't all that positive. It demonstrates that, considering your aerobic ability, you are still capable of running faster. When your MAF is 8 minutes per mile, you should not be able to race a 5 km event in a time that eclipses 20 minutes, or at about a 6:30 pace.

To have the capacity to run faster than your body would normally permit, signals that you are a candidate for injury and/or illness. If your anaerobic capacity is greater than your aerobic capacity, it means you have a chemical imbalance. This kind of dissonance often leads to a physical imbalance which can then traumatize the body.

Swimming

For swimmers — especially those who don't have access to a coach — the HRM is indispensable, because it will encourage them to train harder and more efficiently. Of course, you must make sure you select a HRM that is guaranteed to be waterproof.

Swimming in a pool, a lake, or the ocean, tends to limit gravity's stress on the athlete. The only resistance a swimmer faces is the water itself. The pull of gravity, therefore, is much lower as compared to its effect on land in such activities as running and cycling. Due to this phenomenon, swimmers have to expend a lot of effort to get their heart rate into the target zone. Also, to produce an exceptional performance in the water, a swimmer, like a cyclist, must exhibit a high level of technical proficiency.

MAF-Test for Swimmers

Just as with cycling and running, you can employ the MAF-test to monitor your swimming improvements. An indoor pool at your local Y, club, high school, or college is an excellent place to conduct this examination. Usually, the environment factors — lane distance and temperature — remain constant.

Swimmers have a choice of administering the MAF-test in one of two ways. They can either time themselves over a specified distance — say 1000 yards — or for the number of laps they plan on swimming. Regardless of which procedure is used, it's essential to try to keep the heart rate within the target zone.

It's very simple for swimmers to determine whether or not they are making training progress: After several months of conducting the MAF-test, you should be able to swim the same number of laps — or distance — in faster times at the same heart rate.

Suppose it takes you 12 minutes and 30 seconds to swim twenty 50 yard laps at your maximum aerobic heart rate of 145 bpm when you first start conducting the MAF-test. After a month of adhering to your training regimen, you might be able to cover this same distance — at the same maximum aerobic heart rate — in, say, 12 minutes flat. A month later, it would not be inconceivable for your heart rate to remain at 145 bpm, while your time for these twenty 50 yard laps dropped to 11 minutes and 45 seconds.

By contrast, if your times for this distance become slower, it may be indicative of any one of the following problems: an impending injury and/or illness, overtraining, or too much stress in your living circumstances. Upon ascertaining the cause(s) of your regression, it's essential to make the appropriate revisions. This could mean a modification of your diet, lifestyle, and/or training program.

Anaerobic Intervals and Competition

Novice swimmers who have completed their base training may easily surpass aerobic maximum heart rates when doing anaerobic intervals or engaging in competition. If this is your situation, the HRM will only be beneficial for warming up, cooling down and recovery periods during interval sessions.

Generally, using a HRM during a race is impractical. Looking at the unit while churning through the water would more than likely disrupt the mechanics of swimming. Yet the HRM can be very helpful if you participate in triathlons or several events on the same day. In these cases, the device will help you relax as well as evaluate your heart rate while preparing yourself for the next competitive segment.

Triathlons and Biathlons

Those athletes who become proficient in cycling, running, and swimming can experience the challenge and excitement of multi-sport competition. Usually, a biathlon event follows the sequence of run-bike-run; while a triathlon begins with a swim, then has a bike leg, and concludes with a run. A heart rate monitor can help you do your best in all of these events.

As with other forms of endurance contests, use the monitor to help you warm-up thoroughly. Once the contest gets under way, the device can remind you to maintain your maximum racing heart rate. As mentioned previously, this is a more efficient way of competing than having your pulse rate go through peaks and valleys — which, ultimately, is a waste of energy.

Let's assume, for example, your maximum racing heart rate is 165 bpm. During competition, you don't want to deviate more than 5 bpm above or below that figure. Yet, not only do you feel very good early in the race, but your heart rate is 5 bpm lower than normal. If you are fortunate enough to be in this position, it should provide an incentive to push yourself harder.

Conversely, just after a race begins, you may find yourself in a radically different situation. Along with feeling bad, you may discover that your heart rate is well above the normal target zone. When this happens, it's crucial to slow down. Failure to do so could result in not finishing your event or turning in a sub-par performance.

In order to do well in a triathlon and biathlon, you must make smooth transitions. As you gain experience in these events, you will learn that the key to doing this is staying relaxed. While you rapidly shift from one discipline to another, look at your HRM: It will remind you to breathe deeply and stay calm, which will both conserve energy and bring your heart rate down.

CHAPTER 10

Breathing: The Forgotten Component

When training or competing, all too many athletes fail to consider the way they are breathing. Like their non-athletic counterparts, they merely inhale and exhale in an unconscious manner. What both groups of people don't understand is that their heart rate will rise if they breathe incorrectly.

Is there really a right and a wrong way to breathe? Definitely: Only by breathing in accordance with the following pattern, can you hope to reach optimum health and fitness:

☐ While inhaling, your abdominal muscles should be relaxed and gently pushed out, as you simultaneously extend the spine slightly.

☐ Inhalation calls for pulling in, or contracting, the abdominal muscles, as the spine is slightly flexed forward.

☐ Throughout this process, there is very little chest movement. Only during forced exhalations should the chest expand and, then too, the abdominals must be relaxed and extended (pushed out).

Most people, due to breathing habits developed in early childhood use a breathing technique that is a far cry from this most effective pattern. When inhaling, their abdomen is pulled in and the chest rises; when exhaling, their chest falls and the the abdomen heaves outward. This breathing style has a strong negative by-product: The lungs exchange significantly less air during the inhalation-exhalation process. Over time, this can create a tremendous amount of stress on the body — and such stress becomes especially profound for the athlete while training or competing.

Here is a suggestion that will help you re-learn how to breathe correctly:

☐ While standing, place your right band on the middle of your abdomen. Put the left one on the thoraco-lumbar, i.e. the middle to lower section of the spine. Then slowly breathe in and out. Relax the abdominal muscles, allowing them to fall out on the inhalations and contract on the exhalations. Imagine the space that your hands surround is an empty vessel you are filling with air. Each morning and evening, devote 5–10 minutes to this practice for as long as it takes to get the hang of it.

Learning how to breathe correctly can be inhibited by a weak diaphragm muscle. To determine whether or not you have this problem, see how you do on these three simple self-examinations:

1. Breath Holding Time:
This test accurately measures the diaphragm's general capacity. Take a deep breath and see how long you can hold it. If you are in good health, you should be able to hold your breath for at least 50 seconds.

2. Snider's Test:
Relying on the power of breath, this exam evaluates the diaphragm muscle's strength. Hold a lit match about six inches away from your mouth. With your mouth wide open, try to blow the flame out. If you have the slightest difficulty doing this, certainly a problem may exist.

3. Vital Capacity:

In order to make this assessment, you will need a hand-held spirometer. Although this instrument cannot measure the rate of expired air, it can measure the amount of air (in cubic centimeters) that you can force out of your lungs. This number can be converted into a percentage of normal capacity as it relates to your height. On the spirometer's scale, which tops out at 120 percent, you should register somewhere between 55 and 110 percent. Studies show that Vital Capacity has a direct correlation to a person's physiological age: The lower

---

Case History: Gordon's Energy

In all facets of life, Gordon was extremely disciplined. And he used this quality to get the most out of his bicycle training program. He always wore his HRM, ate the right food and, most importantly, he had carefully analyzed his abilities and objectives. Yet despite this balanced approach to exercising, he did have one significant problem: When competing, he gradually became so fatigued, he never had enough energy during the final miles to be a real threat at the finish line.

A quick observation revealed that Gordon wasn't breathing properly. It was suggested that he reverse his inhalation and exhalation patterns and then perform a series of exercises to strengthen the abdominal muscles. Since Gordon had been breathing incorrectly for 39 years, he initially experienced some difficulty making these adaptations. Yet he took a disciplined approach and mastered this crucial breathing rhythm in less than a month. This not only helped him become a top-ten contender, but it also improved his overall health and fitness.

---

the Vital Capacity, the higher the physiological age, and vice versa.

If you score low on any of these 3 tests, you can strengthen your diaphragm muscle with a simple drill, the *straw exercise*. Place a straw in your mouth and breathe, in the correct pattern, for one or two minutes. Perform this exercise three times per week for two months, gradually working up to several two-minute sets. If you have a weak diaphragm, the straw exercise may prove difficult at first but you will have little trouble doing it after some practice.

Both a stronger diaphragm muscle and the correct breathing technique will make you much more efficient in your athletic endeavors. Your MAF, for example, can dramatically improve from one workout to the next, simply by extending the stomach downward when you take a breath. Another valuable dividend that is gained from breathing correctly is that you will be able to go faster at your normal heart rate.

CHAPTER 11

The Effect of Altitude

Training and competing at altitudes above 3000 ft (1000 m) increases the level of stress on an athlete's body, something that is particularly relevant in cycling. However, using a HRM to tackle an arduous ascent can make this additional stress work *for* rather than against you.

Riding in the mountains is dramatically different from riding at sea level. Not only do you have to work harder, but your breathing also becomes noticeably more difficult. Breathing becomes more of a problem at elevation because the atmospheric pressure is lower in this environment. As a result, the body takes in less oxygen. When this happens, it takes more effort to do the same amount of work — which is indicated by a marked rise in your 'normal' heart rate.

And since most cyclists train by quantity (miles) rather than quality (intensity), their higher heart rates can lead to more injuries — both structural and biochemical — while they are riding at elevation. Frequently, a rider's response to this situation is to become depressed or anxious. In part, this emotional state is due to the increased production of lactic acid associated with the lower oxygen uptake. (It is well known that higher lactic acid levels can trigger such changes in temperament.)

Regrettably, many cyclists who relocate to train in the mountains base this move on a questionable assumption. Originally, it was believed that the body, responding to the decreased oxygen uptake at higher elevations, produced an increased number of red blood cells. It has proven very difficult, however, to assert this hypothesis with absolute certain-

Case History: Brian's Adjustments

Brian, 25, was making incredible progress as a competitive cyclist. In fact, he had rapidly become one of the best racers on the eastern seaboard. Because he was a high school teacher, he could devote his entire summer to training and competing. In order to make some real fitness gains, he decided to head for the mountains, and went to Boulder, Colorado.

This cycling mecca, complete with name riders and awesome landscape, had the desired affect: Brian redoubled his commitment to train harder. With the altitude elevating his heart rate, Brian pushed himself to keep up with the local hot shots. As a result of these two new stresses, he destroyed the healthy state of his mind and body. Brian's leg muscles convulsed with muscle spasms and, unable to ride, he was overcome by depression.

An agonizing telephone conversation with his sports medicine doctor produced the same advice Brian had received before departing: He was reminded to pay close attention to his heart rate readings and stick to the same training program that had produced a high level of achievement before.

After spending three weeks training alone, Brian's health and performance radically improved. Eventually, he rode with pack again — but only during aerobic workouts. On the days that called for anaerobic intervals, Brian either did them by himself or with a couple of riders whose abilities matched his.

Upon returning to the east coast, at the end of the summer, Brian had the kind of race results that most cyclists can only dream about.

ty. A study conducted in 1986 by Dr. Robert Glover at the University of Colorado has raised some fascinating questions about red blood cell production. His research clearly demonstrated that red blood cells do not significantly increase in number when an individual is at high altitudes. Furthermore, Dr. Glover discovered that at elevation, plasma levels are lowered as a result of leakage from circulation. This escaping plasma tends to promote a more concentrated population of red blood cells which, in turn, creates the *appearance* of higher numbers. Still, proper training in the mountains may provide benefits to the cyclist.

To ensure the chances of this occurring, the body must be given a reasonable period to adapt to the added stress of living and riding at altitude. Riders hoping to improve their conditioning, therefore, will have to spend two to three weeks acclimatizing to this new environment. A HRM will remove the guesswork from your adaptation process. By wearing the device both on as well as off the bicycle, you can remain aware of the essential triad of heart rate information: your morning heart rate, your resting pulse rate, and your MAF in the target zone. Initially, all three of these parameters will probably be slightly higher than normal.

The time required for these readings to stabilize depends on your degree of fitness. Upon adjusting to your alpine surroundings, you will begin to make conditioning advances. These improvements, however, will be similar to the gains you can attain at sea level. But should you travel above 10,000 feet, expect to have some trouble making gains in your fitness. At this height, oxygen uptake is dramatically lower than at sea level.

Eventually, after coming down from the mountains, you will have developed a marked increase in your oxygen uptake. Dropping from 1,863 meters to sea level, for example, will increase oxygen uptake by 11.1 percent. A decent of 3,000 meters increases the total oxygen uptake by nearly 18 percent! Corresponding incremental jumps in fitness would usually require many months—or years—of training on a daily basis. Yet, even if all goes well for you while training at altitude, don't expect this kind of change to take place immediately upon descending. It will require about three weeks to achieve such a peak conditioning experience.

To verify any improvements in oxygen uptake, check out your MAF. Racers, in particular, should make careful note of this aforementioned sequence: adaptation, training, descending, and peaking. Failure to accurately account for the days needed to meet this schedule could mean that you won't derive oxygen uptake benefits in time for a specific competition. Remember, just riding at altitude will not automatically enhance your training program. You must pay strict attention to your bodily changes. And when it comes to obtaining this essential information, there's no better tool than a HRM.

CHAPTER 12

Injury and Rehabilitation

Nothing can be more frustrating to a dedicated athlete than sustaining a serious injury or illness that curtails his or her workouts and/or competition. Athletes know all too well that a malady that interferes with their activity for several weeks — or months — will engender a loss of fitness. Often, people faced with this prospect become either mildly depressed or ridden with anxiety.

One of the major underlying themes of this volume is that a HRM, when used correctly, can prevent many sports-related injuries. Moreover, in certain instances, the HRM can be used as a therapeutic device to help you get back on your feet after an injury or illness. And, lastly, it can help you *prevent* common physical maladies.

Many injuries that plague athletes are caused by overtraining. As previously mentioned, this phenomenon can easily be prevented by using a HRM to train in the target zone, and to check your morning and resting pulse levels.

But let's say you are beleaguered by an over-training injury before you start using a HRM. How can you use the device to get your body back on the right track? Simple: As noted in Chapter 2, when computing the target zone numbers, you must take an injury into consideration. Having done that, train within this parameter for two or three weeks. If your injury does not heal within this period, you will have to make two important modifications to facilitate your rehabilitation:

116

☐ Should your injury allow you to exercise — even if just for 20 minutes — modifying the target zone downward (see below) should restore you to good health again. If, on the other hand, you feel aches and pains only when working out for more than an hour, it's crucial not to exceed this limit, as well as to make a target zone readjustment. (Of course, the HRM is not a panacea. If you experience pain

---

Case History: Mark's Intuition

Mark was completely satisfied with his training program. What pleased him most was that for the first time in several years he had been able to ride the entire season totally free of excruciating sciatic pain. Mark attributed this good fortune to paying close attention to his HRM. He became so sensitive to this training partner, that he knew exactly what his pulse rate would be even before looking at the numbers displayed on the receiver.

After three years of daily use, the battery in Mark's HRM finally failed. He decided not to replace this small, inexpensive item but, instead, relied on his intuition to assess his pulse rate.

Within four months of intuitive training, Mark was jolted by a severe sciatic episode. One morning, when the pain in his leg was particularly acute, he called his sports physician to arrange an appointment. Instead of seeing Mark, the doctor offered the following advice: Replace the HRM's battery, lower the target zone range 10 bpm, and then spend a few days on the bike only spinning during workouts.

Two days later, Mark felt no discomfort and was able to resume his normal training regimen.

---

or discomfort the moment you start exercising, this indicates a need to see a heath professional.) For both of the above examples, here is the procedure for the proper heart rate adjustments:

a. Using your present target zone as a guide, employ the lower number as the new high number of the modified range. Then subtract 10 from this lower number to arrive at the new base figure of your target zone.

b. If your normal aerobic training range happens to be 140 bpm to 150 bpm, alter this down to 130–140 for the rehabilitation period. The length of time you should maintain this new target rate will be explained below.

☐ Extend the warm-up and cool-down periods by 50 percent while you are working out in the rehabilitation phase. That means each of the usual 15 minute sessions should be increased to at least 22 minutes. If your regular warm-up and cool-down phases are of longer duration, change both of them accordingly.

Rehabilitation Time Frame

When injured, some athletes tend to adopt a macho attitude. With teeth clinched and a grimace on their face, they will continue training until it truly becomes physically impossible. Others respond to pain and discomfort by becoming overcautious. For them, the mere sight of a blister is a reason to give up.

Both of these psychological dispositions will do little to restore you to a healthy condition. To totally disregard an injury could very well compound its severity. And while rest and relaxation can help the body heal itself, it can be extremely stressful for an athlete to assume a totally inactive stance.

Should you be faced with an injury, be sensible — adopt a middle-of-the-road attitude: Adjust your target zone down, and then proceed with caution.

All athletes experiencing physical problems invariably ask the same question: How long will it take me to get better? The time frame for the restoration of health, obviously, varies with each case. Still, here is a general guideline: After revising the target zone to its rehabilitation range, begin exercising at that level for no more than 3 weeks. Resume training at the normal aerobic heart rate if there is a noticeable improvement at end of this period. Assuming that a relapse of any kind does not occur, you can continue with your regular training program.

Unfortunately, sometimes the rehabilitation process will not go so smoothly. Upon returning to the normal target zone, the injury may flare up again, leading to a disappointing regression. Don't lose heart: Immediately change the target zone back to its rehabilitation parameters and train at that level for another 3 weeks. Sometimes, this aerobic modification period still won't do the trick. When that happens, continue in this modified zone for another 3 weeks.

If you are not improving — or feeling worse — after this 6-week rehabilitation segment, you should consult a health professional.

Preventing and Recovering from Illness

Even the most finely tuned athletic 'machine' may come down with sniffles, a cold or the flu. When this happens, your body's metabolism increases to fight off and recover from this annoying or disabling invader. Usually, the struggle for the restoration of good health will raise your normal heart rate.

If you do notice a rise in your resting and active pulse rates, it's best to stop working out for one or two days. Failure to do so could lower your body's defenses and allow the illness to get a good grip on your system.

Should your ailment be accompanied by a fever, definitely don't exercise. When your temperature rises above 98.6°F (37°C), your metabolism is racing and, therefore, your heart rate will be elevated. You can resume training as soon as you

---

Case History: Judy's Overtraining Injury

For the third consecutive year, Judy had a great competitive cycling season. But there was one problem: For the first time, an injury forced her to miss a race. Worse still, her next race — an important event at the end of her race calendar — proved to be disastrous from a performance standpoint.

To rectify this shattering race result, Judy trained harder over the winter. By spring, she was in excellent shape — but her injuries reappeared, and she was unable to participate in any early season contests.

It was recommended that Judy devote four months to building a solid aerobic base. She was reluctant to follow this advice because she didn't want to spend so much time doing only 'easy' training rides. In the end, since she had run out of options, she decided to go along with the base-building program.

By early summer Judy's endurance and aerobic speed had improved significantly. In her first criterium, which marked the beginning of the anaerobic phase of training, she performed much better than she had hoped for. Throughout the summer, Judy's race results continued to improve and by the end of October she was eager to begin her long base period.

---

are fever-free for 24 hours and your morning heart rate is within 3 beats of its normal reading.

After getting back to training, you may feel good enough to perform a strenuous workout. Resist this temptation. Remember, your body is still in the recuperative phase from an illness. To jump aggressively back into your training routine could cause a serious relapse. The way to avoid this possibility is to spend two or three days exercising with your target zone reduced by 10 bpm. So, if your regular range is 135–145, reduce the span to 125–135. This conservative approach should bring your morning heart rate down to normal, which indicates that you're ready to train hard again.

Although these remedial procedures are simple enough, some athletes will not adopt them for fear that a couple of days resting, or at least not going full blast, will provide their competitors with an edge. Ultimately, a more serviceable approach harmonizes the desire for peak conditioning and the need for good health.

CHAPTER 13

Conclusion

'Even the longest journey begins with the first step,' states the Tao Te Ching, the Chinese book of proverbs. The first step, then, to improving both your health and fitness is taking the time to exercise regularly. In order to sustain a high level of enthusiasm, here are some simple suggestions to follow.

First, establish realistic objectives. There are numerous reasons to start an exercise program — becoming fitter, losing weight, or becoming the first person on your block to win the New York marathon or the Tour de France's yellow jersey. Regardless of your avowed purpose, take an objective look at your circumstances. If you're 6 ft 4 and tip the scales at 250 pounds, it's highly unlikely that you'll become a 'King of the Mountains.' Moreover, at age 45, don't expect to develop the cardiovascular capacity of Ironman Mark Allen or Tour de France victor Greg Lemond. And even if you are 19 years old and in phenomenal shape, your chances of defeating a world-class athlete are ever so slight.

All this is not to say that you shouldn't bring high aspirations to your training program. However, it's advisable to be ruthlessly honest with yourself about the physical material you are working with. Just remember, you can reach your full athletic potential and become healthier by consistently working out with a HRM.

Still, some athletes become so obsessed with becoming fitter and winning races, they create conflicts at home, at school, or in the workplace. Before designing and committing yourself to an exercise program, consider how it will effect your primary obligations. A well conceived training and/or competition agenda should not interfere with your daily existence.

Second, maintain a diary. Each day, take the time to record the following information: your morning pulse, high and low heart rates for each training or competitive event, and a few comments that characterize your performance (the type of activity, times, placing, how you felt). These notations will provide you with invaluable data about your progress, plateaus, as well as regressions. By carefully analyzing this record, you can make the necessary adjustments that will promote your overall well-being.

Third, when training, discard the anachronistic athletic axiom 'No Pain, No Gain.' Upon the completion of an aerobic workout that has been performed correctly, you should feel like you have enough energy to perform it again — immediately. If you finsh a training session feeling totally wasted, chances are you have been overexerting yourself. Although this intense effort can raise your pain threshold, the fundamental purpose of exercising is to preserve a bodily balance between health and fitness.

Both health and conditioning are clearly lifelong endeavors. Still, each day that you train will generate immediate benefits. Not only will you look and feel better, but you will also have a more energy, as well as the capacity to be more productive. These worthwhile goals are clearly attainable by working out with a heart rate monitor.

Appendix: Heart Rate Monitor Contacts

Ciclo Sport USA
1540 1E Barclay Blvd.
Buffalo Grove, IL 60089
Tel: (800) 279-2820

Computer Instruments Corporation
100 Madison Ave.
Hempstead, NY 11550
(516) 483-8200

Elexis Corporation
7000 NW 46th St.
Miami, FL 33166
(305) 592-6069

Nike
9000 SW Nimbus
Beaverton, OR 97005
(503) 644-9000

Polar USA
470 West Ave
Stamford, CT 06902
(800) 262-7776

Precise International
15 Corporate Drive
Orangeburg, NY 10962
(800) 431-2996

Schwinn Bicycle Company
217 N Jefferson St.
Chicago, IL 60606
(312) 454-7400

BIBLIOGRAPHY

General Reading:

Baily, Covert. *Fit or Fat*. Boston, MA: Houghton Mifflin, 1977.

Borysewics, Edward. *Bicycle Road Racing*. Brattleboro, VT: Vitesse Press, 1985.

Conconi, Francesco. *Moser's Hour Records: A Human and Scientific Adventure*. (Translated by Patricia Ennis). Brattleboro, VT: Vitesse Press, 1991.

Maffetone, Philip. *Everyone is an Athlete*. Mahopac, NY: Barmore Productions, 1990.

Technical Reading:

Conconi, Francesco, et al. "Determination of the Anaerobic Threshold by a Noninvasive Field Test in Runners." *Cattedra di Biochemica Applicata*. Ferrera, Italy:1980.

Janssen, Peter G. J. M. *Training Lactate Pulse Rate*. Polar Electro Oy, Finland, 1998. (Dr. Janssen has worked with two Dutch professional cycling teams, Panasonic and PDM. He is an advocate of the Conconi training method and his book, while excellent, is extremely technical.)

Landoni. *Agnostic Cycling*. Milan, Italy: Arti Grafiche (undated).

McArdle, W. D. *Exercise Physiology*. Philadelphia: Lae and Febrger, 1986.

Index

List of Titles Available from Bicycle Books

Title	Author	US Price
The Mountain Bike Book	Rob van der Plas	$9.95
The Bicycle Repair Book	Rob van der Plas	$8.95
The Bicycle Racing Guide	Rob van der Plas	$10.95
The Bicycle Touring Manual	Rob van der Plas	$10.95
Roadside Bicycle Repairs	Rob van der Plas	$4.95
Major Taylor (hardcover)	Andrew Ritchie	$19.95
Bicycling Fuel	Richard Rafoth	$7.95
In High Gear (hardcover)	Samuel Abt	$21.95
In High Gear (paperback)	Samuel Abt	$10.95
Mountain Bike Maintenance	Rob van der Plas	$7.95
The Bicycle Fitness Book	Rob van der Plas	$7.95
The Bicycle Commuting Book	Rob van der Plas	$7.95
The New Bike Book	Jim Langley	$4.95
Tour of the Forest Bike Race	H. E. Thomson	$9.95
Bicycle Technology	Rob van der Plas	$16.95
Tour de France (hardcover)	Samuel Abt	$22.95
Tour de France (paperback)	Samuel Abt	$12.95
LeMond (not available in UK)	Samuel Abt	$18.95
All Terrain Biking	Jim Zarka	$7.95
Mountain Bike Magic	Rob van der Plas	$14.95
The High Performance Heart	Maffetone/Mantell	$9.95

Buy our books at your local book shop or bike store.
Book shops can obtain these titles for you from our book trade distributor (listed on the copyright page) and the major national and regional wholesalers. Bike shops can order them directly from us. If you have difficulty obtaining our books elsewhere, we will be pleased to supply them by mail, but we must add $2.50 postage and handling (as well as California Sales Tax if mailed to a California address). Prepayment by check (or credit card information) must be included with your order.

Bicycle Books, Inc.
PO Box 2038
Mill Valley CA 94941
Tel.: (415) 381-0172

In Britain: Bicycle Books
463 Ashley Road
Poole, Dorset BH14 0AX
Tel.: (0202) 71 53 49